The Seattle Sutton Solution

No Gimmicks

by

Seattle Sutton

ISBN: 0-9752784-052995

Printed in the United States
By ADventure Printing
Ottawa, Illinois

Cover photograph by Jim Luning
Cover photograph

Dedicated to family past, present, and future. Especially my husband, mother, father, children and their spouses, grandchildren, grandparents, aunts, uncles, nieces, nephews, dear sisters. These I know. To them and family yet unknown, launching from thc power of this eternal moment, I send greetings and love rippling through time fore and time aft.

Happiness.

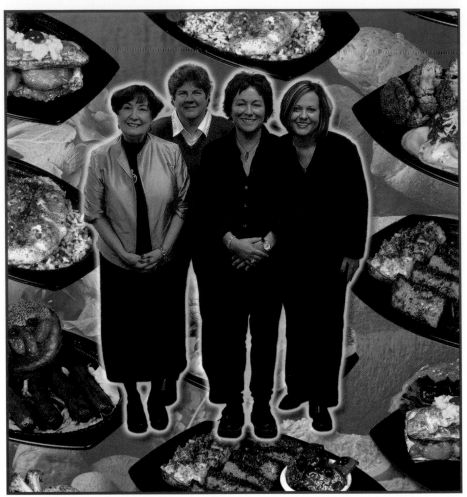

Seattle Sutton, Kathleen Tuntland, Ruth Egofske, Sarah Borgstrom

"To be clear, let me say that all four owners very much like and admire men. We're all happily married. We're not militant feminists. We love our husbands, though we often sit back and laugh about the fact we don't believe that they—or maybe any other four men—could have grown our business and made a success like we have."

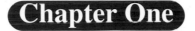

Chapter One

The Bible says, "To those whom much is given, much is expected." I believe every single human being inherently possesses at least one unique and helpful trait.

I was born with energy to burn…and have been relentlessly igniting it for more than seventy-two years. Thank goodness—with appropriate fuel—human energy is continuously renewable.

Healthy eating. The right fuel. Healthy living. The happy result.

I'm not one to bury the lead, as they say in the news profession. So here's my primary message, the core essence of this book, presented to you in the fourth paragraph of the first chapter: "Exercise your thinking rights. Choose wisely. Live happily."

What is happiness? Doesn't your answer reflect one of the beauties of freedom?

We are free to think. We are free to choose. We don't do either in a vacuum. We balance faith and fear, ambition and inertia, confidence and insecurity, strength and weakness, belief and doubt. We consider family, friends, and our connection with the web of life.

The "web of life" is an expression credited to my namesake, Chief Seattle. It means we're all part of the same whole…an aggregate greater than its sum.

All things considered, I agree. My sense of the reality of such a web has been a reliable guide to help me make choices and handle their consequences.

Remembering my life—re-living it in a real way, in order to write it down—has been a singular and invigorating pleasure. Looking back, I am able to diagram how my earlier thoughts and experiences led me to design and build a company that prepares and delivers fresh and healthy meals.

Fascinating. The philosopher Arthur Schopenhauer had the opinion that every life, viewed in retrospect, is arranged like a good novel. Or, I might add, an intriguing movie.

And here's the most exciting part: I couldn't help but notice that, while I am living mine, I am also writing it. This is not unique to me.

Your life, for example, is your movie. You are the star, the scriptwriter, the director, and the producer. Meeting those responsibilities requires a lot of energy. Which brings us back to fuel.

What we eat is, by definition, our diet. So everyone is on a diet.

You are reading a book about healthy eating. Therefore, it is a diet book. The last one you'll ever need, in my opinion, because Seattle Sutton's Healthy Eating is based on common sense and scientific fact.

The shaping events of my life, and my desire to improve people's eating habits, have been intertwined for decades. Here are a few examples:

Scene One:

During my childhood years, people didn't read food labels, didn't think much about what they were eating, didn't know much about calories. My dear father, so wonderful to me all our lives together, kept gaining weight until eventually he tipped the scales at 385 pounds. When I went away to nursing school in 1950, I worried so much about him that I mailed menu plans for my mother to follow.

His doctors told him to lose 100 pounds or face the certain prospect of congestive heart failure. To shed his excess, he tried hard to minimize his food intake. Despite some temporary success, he was unable to overcome the frustrations of maintaining a "gimmick" diet.

Scene Two:

In 1969, when our children had grown, I began to assist my husband in his medical practice in Marseilles, Illinois (about 70 miles southwest of Chicago). Kelly was a true family doctor. He did it all—obstetrics, pediatrics, orthopedics. There were no specialists around when he began his practice in 1957.

Some people tease me that I married Kelly Sutton because my first name went so well with his last. Whatever prompted our nuptials should be praised, because in August of 2004, we celebrate our 50th wedding anniversary.

Much of my time in Dr. Sutton's office was devoted to paperwork and administrative matters. I learned quite a bit about the practicalities of managing a business.

I was also involved with his patients. Knowing of my strong interest in helping the obese improve their nutrition, Kelly asked me to educate them about healthy eating.

How discouraging to hand patients a piece of paper listing foods to eat and avoid, knowing they most likely would not follow the guidelines.

I'm a nurse! I want to heal! I ached to find a better way!

Scene Three:

Quite a few years later, in 1985, Kelly was treating a Type 2 diabetes patient named Rodney Juergensen. Rodney listened while I outlined a healthy diet. He seemed attentive, but not enthusiastic.

Finally, he sighed, and looked me in the eye. "I know I should do what you suggest, but I am certain I won't. But I will follow your plan if you cook the meals for me."

In a flash the whole idea for Seattle Sutton's Healthy Eating—in its entirety—came to me. I realized how to give people what they needed…how to plan…how to prepare…how to deliver.

Everything coalesced in one bright and shining instant. In a book or movie, they call such an event the "hinge."

My "hinge" was like a burning bush. We all have the potential for such a moment. Of course I had been preparing—without knowing it virtually my whole life. That's the movie I am making.

Oh, sure, there was work to do. Plenty! But now I had the blueprint in my head. How should I begin? Here's a quote by an ancient Chinese sage that describes the process:

Lao Tzu: "Undertake difficult tasks by approaching what is easy in them; do great deeds by focusing on their minute aspects."

Beginning with just a few customers, progressing step-by-step, Seattle Sutton's Healthy Eating has slowly advanced for nearly twenty years. We figured out a healthy menu plan, designed a mass-production kitchen, built our own truck-line. We learned how to soak your beans, bake your muffins, roast your turkey, and we deliver our meals to you fresh.

Our first week (in 1985), our total order was 231 meals, mostly within or near Marseilles. In 2004, Seattle Sutton's Healthy Eating prepared and delivered as many as 150,000 meals a week to customers in Illinois, Indiana, Wisconsin, Iowa, Michigan, Minnesota, Nebraska, and Georgia.

Our customers, if they're honest with the program, lose weight and maintain their loss. Many have dropped more than 100 pounds. One man lost 215 pounds, and has maintained his new weight. The usual pace is one to three pounds a week, until a goal is reached.

All this without having to resort to unhealthy gimmick diets. In the following pages, I'll have a lot to say about fake or ill-considered weight loss schemes foisted on the public by business people overly concerned with gaining wealth and fame.

Let me give you a preliminary summation: Weight is gained or lost according to a basic calculation of calories in vs. calories out.

Common sense and truth.

Our meals provide many benefits, not limited to weight reduction. Type 2 diabetics do very well. I give you as an example a 75-year old diabetic from Waukegan, Illinois, who lost 105 pounds eating our meals, and was able to stop using diabetic medication for the first time in 40 years.

Senior citizen customers can extend their years of independent living because we take care of every aspect of meal preparation. Often, it is an inability to shop and cook that hastens the necessity of leaving the sanctuary of home.

Some of our customers, who may not need to lose weight, stay on our program because of a desire to eat healthy, and an appreciation of our program's convenience.

A person's greatest asset is not a house, or a car, or money in a bank. It's good health, and to keep it, we must make smart decisions. If we smoke, we should stop. If we ride in a car, we should wear a seat belt. If we lift a fork to our mouth, it should be hoisting healthy food.

When you eat right, you're fueling right, and when you're fueling right, you're feeling right. When you're feeling right, you have the energy to think right and do right. That's the path to happiness.

By the way, Seattle Sutton's Healthy Eating is a company mostly owned by women. Our business values can be accurately described as: good listening, patience, compassion, problem solving, nurturing, openness, and trust.

Hardly the dog-eat-dog doctrine. You know—the philosophy of people who run companies like Enron, and World Com (MCI), and Arthur Anderson.

We are grossing almost 19 million dollars a year now, and growing at an average annual rate of approximately 20%, with no end in sight.

And why not? In our modern world, people have neither the time nor the inclination to use the kitchen. Seattle Sutton's Healthy Eating brings nutrition to your table, like a good mother.

To paraphrase Pat and Barbara McDonald, "Our future's so bright, we have to wear shades."

I also believe that—under the guidance of four women—the people of our company have built a new model for American business, based on ideas more commonly found in small towns, where folks are less inclined to an excess of greed and unnecessary selfish confrontation.

In the following pages, I take the presumptive liberty of attempting to communicate what are called (often derisively) small town values, seeking to demonstrate their relevance and application in our contemporary world, particularly in reference to how we eat, and how we can be happier.

Intermittently throughout this book, after chapters 2, 4, 6, 8, 10, 12, 14, and 16, I'm going to step away from the biography and insert a few of my ideas about nutrition and diets. By presenting healthy eating do's and don'ts in such a fashion, I hope to more strongly emphasize their importance.

In the same sections, I will include witness and testimony from people who have benefited from our meal replacement program.

Anyone, of course, can provide testimonials, and if they do not exist, some are willing to invent them. I promise that you will read the real words of real people who have reaped real benefits, and are enthusiastically proud to represent their true situations and opinions.

My life, my business, and my ideas about nutrition are all interrelated. My book tells the truth about all three, as I know it. You have my word.

I'm so pleased to give it, because I wholeheartedly concur with Ralph Waldo Emerson, who said: "Don't worry about the consequences of honesty."

Here is another quote, with which I wish to close Chapter One.

Logan Pearsall Smith: "There are two things to aim at in life: first, to get what you want; and, after that, to enjoy it. Only the wisest...achieve the second."

Chapter Two

My ancestors migrated to America from Germany by way of Russia, constantly seeking the opportunity to live free and secure a harvest proportional to their labor. Their lives, like ours, were full of challenges.

We finally found our fair home, not in Western or Eastern Europe, but in the United States, in North Dakota, in and around the village of Gackle.

I was born a Remboldt. My family lived on a small farm several miles from Gackle. Grandmother Remboldt was a mid-wife who delivered practically everybody in the neighborhood, including me, my older sister (by a year) Aleaine, and my younger sisters, May and June, who were twins.

My grandfather wanted to name me. He bribed my parents by offering to give me his favorite quilt. They probably would have said yes to him without the gift, but I'm glad they allowed it. I loved that tasseled orange quilt, especially because my grandfather sacrificed it for me. I still remember using it as a playground for my dolls.

At the time of my birth, my grandfather was reading a newspaper article about the Indian Chief Seattle. So, even though I'm not Native American, I received my name in somewhat the same manner an Indian maiden might receive hers. That is, her family associates her with something that happens at the time of her birth.

Two years later, on a typically cold January day in North Dakota, the twins were born. They were premature, as can happen with twinning. My family worked hard to keep the babies warm, simulating the effects of an incubator by heating bricks on the coal stove, and placing them in the twin's little bed, which my father had made from boxes.

There was no doctor. Grandma Remboldt and my mother worked tirelessly, but my sisters didn't survive. One lived seven hours, and the other, seven days. My dad handmade their coffins.

Where have they been these last seventy years? Somewhere beautiful, I'm quite sure.

My mother came from a family of 16, including two sets of twins. My dad had six siblings. Which gave me a lot of cousins. Our own family—only two children—was quite small in comparison.

My years as a toddler on the farm were very satisfying, though I experienced the wonder of the feeling long before the actual word "satisfied" entered my vocabulary. My dad and mom were natural born experts in generating love and self-confidence. I don't ever remember a time when I didn't feel I could achieve my goals. What greater gifts could parents possibly give?

The depression came down in full force during my childhood. I had no frame of reference to help me distinguish between easy and hard times, but I do remember how much the family worried about coyotes getting into our chicken coop. We could hear their threatening howls, especially at night.

Our chickens were valuable to us. We could eat their eggs and their flesh. We couldn't afford to lose even one to a wild predator.

The farm also supported a milking herd. Our smart dog, Mopes, had a sense of time (perhaps cued by the sun's position in the sky), and knew when to go out and round up the cattle. Mopes did this every single afternoon, all by himself. We never had to prompt him.

Old clothes were never thrown away. My mother cut out the best parts and used them to make quilts and blankets.

Quilting get-togethers were an important part of social life in and around Gackle. Someone brought big quilting sticks, and everyone pitched in, visiting and enjoying each other's company while working.

Unselfish work was an essential element of our play. We cherished the moment the completed quilt was presented to one of our participating families.

Similarly, we might gather on a Saturday—the men wielding carpentry tools and the women providing food and water—to help a neighbor build a barn.

I wonder if you have experienced the exquisite satisfaction—I hope so—of working with friends in this way. Both quilting and barn-raising represent a perfect alignment of community intent, conscience, and action, and are a powerful antidote against psychological or economic darkness.

I did not perceive our family as poor. My parents—and grandparents—never suggested that we lived in poverty. I thought the whole world existed like we did. Since we were happy. I assumed the same was true for everyone. Shouldn't it be?

We are often frustrated and puzzled that the answer to this question seems to be no, when our heart tells us it should be yes. Regardless, we should never stop trying to put more happiness in the mix.

Our main form of entertainment was going to church or visiting our neighbors. Sometimes they came to see us. We didn't have a phone, so we couldn't call. We simply decided, for example, "Well, tonight let's go visit the Kriegers."

We would harness the horse to the sleigh, and off we would go. I suppose it could have happened that the Kriegers might decide to visit us the same night we did them, and we might miss each other on the trip, and both arrive at an empty house. But it never did.

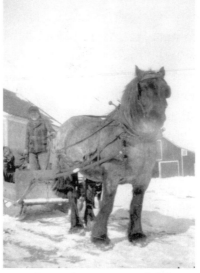

A one horse open sleigh

When we got together, adults would "visit" and children would play. Our favorite game was hide and seek. Sooner or later we'd open the furnace door, insert our wire shaker basket, and make popcorn.

One night we were playing hide and seek at Krieger's farm. They had no electricity (just like us), but many kerosene lamps, one of which caught my sister's hair on fire. Dad had to give her an emergency haircut, which sure looked funny.

Fire accidents notwithstanding, we always had fun. The era's name might have been "the depression," but none of us were emotionally depressed.

But as I grew older, I began to understand the toll that the depression had taken on North Dakota. A persistent drought that lasted half a decade wasn't a positive either. The combination threatened to destroy everything my family had built since my grandparents had arrived in America.

The threat didn't make us cut and run. Remboldts and Zenkers do not wilt under pressure. Neither do most Americans. You do not fold when you are rooted in a place which is your last and best hope.

Everyone worked hard. Harder than ever, actually. Yet the crops were puny and the yield was sparse. We survived by being clever…and wasting nothing. Here's an example: Uncle Bill made wine out of the least edible portions of beets. Beet wine!

Uncle Ben, on the other hand, specialized in homemade beer brewed by placing a mixture of grain, water, and yeast in a warm spot behind the stove.

After a week or two, Ben would retrieve the covered pot, and proudly bottle his own brand. It had a strong beer taste, or maybe that was the yeast. Nobody knew the difference.

My mother didn't know much about balanced meals, but she did know the value of vegetables and fruit. Every fall, she canned them to insure their year round availability.

We didn't have a lot of fresh fruit until it came into season. Our farm had an apple orchard, and Mom was amazingly creative with its fruit. Highly imaginative! Always something healthy. By cleverness, she made the fruit of her labor stretch through an entire year.

Once in a while my mother bought a watermelon at the store in Gackle, as a special treat for the family. We were never able to successfully grow one in our garden. Mother made good use of every portion of a melon, including the rind, which she sliced and pickled.

After my mother baked a cake, she cleaned the bowl so thoroughly during the baking that there appeared to be no need to wash it. It was spotless! She didn't waste a drop of cake batter.

Of course, she still insisted on cleaning the bowl in the sink. She is a Zenker, after all. The Zenkers are very, very clean.

They are also ambitious, in the best sense of the word. If you don't work hard, and you're a Zenker, you're really denounced. You have to give full effort. I'm proud to a Zenker.

The Zenker philosophy is a good one. The Zenkers and the Remboldts, and many others like us, were homesteaders. It's an opportunity to be a landowner, and create a better life. But you have to earn it, and to do so, you can't be stingy with your labor. Many of my first cousins are still farming the same acreage—their very own land!

But work isn't everything. There has to be a balance.

Mom and Dad tended the fields, and milked the cows. Mom separated the cream from the milk, and made our own cottage cheese and butter.

When my mother and father were children, their families hauled wheat to a nearby village—Kulm—and had it milled into flour, a staple of our meals. They stored the flour in the attic of the summer kitchen—a separate building from the main house. Quite a chore to lug the heavy bags.

Mom remains an expert noodle-maker to this day, though she is now more than 93 years old.

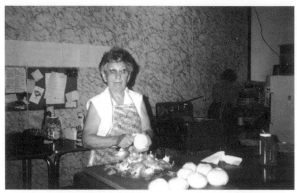

My mother, Alida Zenker Remboldt

Mother made all of our clothes on a treadle Singer sewing machine. She only had one pattern…and it was basic. Since clothes were handed down—child to child and family to family—until they wore out, one was sufficient. Specialized patterns were far too expensive. I never saw her buy or use one.

I had older cousins, and often received dresses from them. I knew that my outgrown ones were passed along as needed.

After all, a girl really only needed two dresses—one for church and one for school. We wore overalls at home.

No one ever said: "I'm tired of that dress."

My mother used her Singer often. Every week, she spent hours mending. Material was studiously recycled. If something was too worn to mend, the bad spot would be cut out, and the remainder used for a doll outfit, or a little doll blanket, or a rug, or whatever.

Mom has been so creative. When we moved into town and got settled, she liked to buy discarded dolls at garage sales in Gackle. She'd take the dolls home, shampoo their hair, and make clothes for them. Think maybe she remembered growing up in a family of fourteen children?

Our prairie home didn't have any running water or indoor toilets. We didn't have a washing machine. And, as I mentioned, we didn't have electricity.

The upstairs of our farmhouse had no direct heat source. Thank goodness warm air rises, and the lignite coal kitchen stove burned well into the night, so we weren't completely unprotected. Besides, Dad usually rose in the "wee hours" and reloaded the stove—really the first "chore" of the day.

We slept on and under homemade goose feather ticks (blankets). Yes, the geese on our farm were important.

Mom and Dad also gave us a rubber hot water bottle. Every cold night, Aleaine and I drew water from the well, heated it on the blessed stove, filled the rubber bottle, and used it to warm the bed.

Even though a dictionary-writer might use a North Dakota winter night to illustrate the meaning of the word "freezing," I don't remember being especially cold. Except in the morning, of course, when I had to get ready for school.

My sister and I ran downstairs and huddled near the stove. One of the real pleasures of childhood was being absolutely certain my parents would have the fire burning. Aleaine and I relied on it.

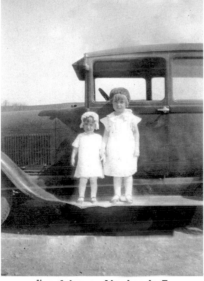

I'm 4 here, Aleaine is 5

We were still living in the country when it came time for me to begin my education. I had a lot to learn, because I didn't yet speak English.

My sister and I walked the two miles each way to the one-room school where eight grades were taught. Of course, in the olden days, miles were a lot longer than they are now. Not really! It just seemed that way.

We carried our lunch, usually a potato apiece. We grew as many as possible, and kept them from freezing by storing them in our root cellar.

The teacher allowed us to place our spud on the coal stove in the middle of the room so it could bake while we were busy with our lessons.

I liked the teacher, whose name was Jack Lang. He boarded with our family, paying $11 per month for room and board. His presence was quite an educational advantage, giving him extra opportunities to tutor me in English and other subjects.

When the weather turned really cold (reminder: we lived in North Dakota where the most reliable forecast guideline is "The North Wind Will Blow And We Shall Have Snow"), my dad hooked our horse, Tony, to the sleigh and dropped us off at school. He returned to pick us up at the end of the day. Some older kids rode their own horses and stabled them in a nearby barn.

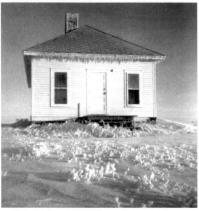

The country school my Mom attended

One of our favorite games revolved around that barn. Literally.

At recess, we played a game called "Ante Over," which involved throwing a ball to the team on the other side of the barn. Once the other kids had the ball, they tried to sneak around and hit us with it. Waiting for them to make their move was very suspenseful.

Many Saturday nights the family made a six-mile trek into Gackle. Mom tucked us into the back of the sleigh, and covered us with feather ticks. The only parts of us anyone could see were our eyes, and the only parts of the universe in our view as we glided across fields of ice and snow were endless layers of Milky Way stars glowing brightly in the dark of night and the black of space.

Most everyone found their way into town on Saturdays. Women shopped for basics, and we all socialized on Main Street, where the children played.

Somewhere around 1940 Hollywood found Gackle. I remember so well the fascination of going into a theater to view enchanting shadows acting out beguiling stories on that big, big screen.

Gone With The Wind. Casablanca. Fantasia. Citizen Kane.

Maybe these were the first times I truly realized that the entire world was not the same as Gackle.

My allowance was two cents a week. My goodness, that bought me a large bag of candy. I know what you're thinking. Sugar! Well, later I'll have some kind words to say about sugar.

I vividly remember one time I couldn't receive my allowance. We had just gotten our first car and were driving it to Gackle, carrying a large can of cream to market. But my dad went round a curve—perhaps a little too fast—and the can tipped over! I might as well say our grocery money tipped over. A genuine tragedy! We cinched our belts tighter that week.

Noodles!

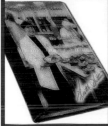

Where's Chapter Three?

It'll be along soon enough. Please let me explain. As I indicated in the first chapter, I'm going to include a few things in the book that don't fit naturally into the flow of the story. So I've prepared eight eight-page insert sections that focus on nutrition.

These sections contain illustrative color photographs and helpful information, including SSHE menus, a recipe for our famous Taco Pie, testimonials from clients of Seattle Sutton's Healthy Eating, and essays on healthy eating titled, "Use Your Thinking Rights."

In preparing these essays, I have drawn on our company's expertise to present you with the very latest that science, experience, and common sense have to say about nutrition. I am particularly grateful for the help of Laura Farjood, a registered dietician who works with our company.

Here are the "Use Your Thinking Rights" topics:
After Chapter 2:
Healthy Eating; Fast Food; Genetics & Obesity.
After Chapter Four:
Mother and Child; Obese Children; Truth About Sugar; Truth About Salt.
After Chapter 6:
Fad & Gimmick Diets; Truth About Fat; Low Carb Diets.
After Chapter 8:
Healthy Eating & Weight Loss; Thin Is Not In; Cheating; Portion Management.
After Chapter 10:
Diet & Diabetes; Disease & Obesity; Depression; Healthy Eating After a Heart Attack.
After Chapter 12:
Supplements, Vitamins, Herbs; Promotional Studies & Genuine Food Science; Organic Foods.
After Chapter 14:
Willpower; Death Foods; Alcohol; Senior Citizens.
After Chapter 16:
Healthy Eating in Schools; Attention School Boards.

So after chapters 2, 4, 6, 8, 10, 12, 14, and 16—eight times in all—we'll insert an eight page section. Following each insert, we'll return to the story.

All right. Here we go. We begin with the first installments of "Use Your Thinking Rights," followed by the menus for Week One of "Seattle Sutton's Healthy Eating" five-week plan.

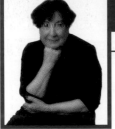

We are what we eat. A well-balanced person eats a well-balanced diet.

Your diet—good or bad—is nothing more or less than the food and drink you consume. A diet rich in fruits, vegetables, whole grains, dairy products, and lean meats may significantly increase longevity and reduce the risk of dying from such illnesses as cancer, heart disease, and stroke.

Eggs can be healthy. Potatoes have a lot of nutritional value. Be careful what you put on them. Count your calories because calories count. Manage your portions.

A pound of body fat contains 3,500 calories. If you eat 100 calories a day more than you expend, you will gain at least ten pounds in a year. Guaranteed! Imagine what happens if you eat 500 extra!

I received a call one day from a lady who told me she couldn't eat any cheese. "It clogs my arteries," she informed me, because she had heard that cheese was binding, and believed whatever she ate went directly into her bloodstream.

In a similar vein (no pun intended), many people believe that when you eat protein it goes right to your muscle. Of course, that's not true.

In fact, protein is not the best energy provider. Most long distance runners prefer to eat carbohydrates instead of protein before a race. They eat pasta, rice, and potatoes.

Good energy foods. Carbohydrates.
Use your thinking rights. Analyze your diet.
Learn facts. Face facts.
Don't be swayed by advertising campaigns.
Is your food good for you? Is it healthy? Or is it habit?
Is your diet energizing you? Or slowing you down?
Helping you? Or killing you?
Go to the mirror. Look into your eyes. Answer honestly.

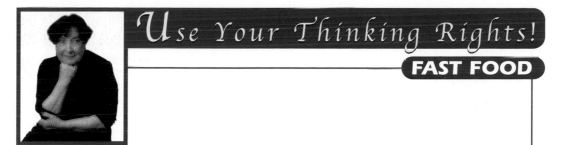

Fast food is okay to eat once in awhile, but it too easily becomes a bad habit, and therefore a real health danger.

Even though many fast food franchises are at long last making efforts to provide "healthier" alternatives, the preparation fundamentals of their approach make this difficult, if not impossible.

A recent study of young Americans (aged 4 to 19) found that one-third of them eat fast food at least once daily. This translates to approximately six pounds of unnecessary additional weight every year.

The study's lead author, Dr. David Ludwig, director of the obesity program at Children's Hospital in Boston, said these results are not a surprise, "since billions of dollars are spent each year on fast-food advertising directed at kids."

The negative effects of too much fast food are cumulative. Seeds of future illness—negatively impacting the length and quality of a life—are being planted.

Children—and parents—are not able to perceive immediate negative effects. Negative health consequences are invisible—for a while.

The power of advertising, the lure of toys and other prizes, and the convenience of the drive-through window combine to make fast food an easy choice for a busy family.

But parents trying to do the right thing for children must realize and meet a basic responsibility. The child is learning how and what to eat. It's important to find and plan healthy meal alternatives that minimize a child's fast food experience. I don't say never, but keep it to a rare occasion, rather than a regular event.

Use your thinking rights! When your children clamor for fast food, it may seem easier to say yes. But no is usually the better answer.

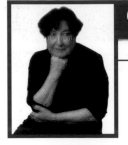

Do some of us have a gene which dooms its possessors to be overweight? I refuse to accept such an inevitability.

Oh, I believe genetics is relevant. Environment isn't everything.

But genetic research is still a toddler science. Identifying an individual gene with the certainty of obesity is quite a stretch given what geneticists now know, though its presence may reasonably indicate a propensity.

When people are able to blame family inheritance for their obesity, they feel powerless, and don't even try to reduce their excess weight.

I think it's more relevant to realize that families pass down their traditions of food choices and overeating. That's what has to be changed. Lifestyle.

So even if you possess the "obesity" gene, refrain from the temptation of using it as a "disabling" excuse to allow yourself to quit trying. You still can make good nutritional decisions. You still have free choice.

A genetic tendency to be obese can be defeated. One can still lose pounds and maintain a lower weight. The reason is just as scientific as genetic research.

Simply put, nutritional science knows, without the possibility of doubt, that weight gain is the result of energy intake in excess of energy use. I preach this constantly. Calories in versus calories out.

Science isn't our only witness. Common sense tells us that eating less and being more active will solve most obesity problems. If you have to work harder to overcome a genetic tendency, isn't it worth it?

Use your thinking rights.

Overcome your genes and fit into smaller jeans.

Sorry! Couldn't resist!

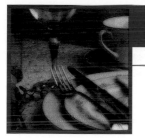

MONDAY:

<u>Dinner:</u> FLUFFY EGG NOODLES WITH MEATBALLS

Seattle Sutton's delicious adaptation of a favorite German noodle dish made with seasoned meatballs in a blended cheese sauce mixed with peas and pimentos over a bed of fluffy noodles.

TUESDAY:

<u>Breakfast:</u> DELIGHTFUL POPPYSEED BREAD & CREAM CHEESE

With chunky applesauce.

<u>Lunch:</u> MOZZARELLA BAKE

An exciting lunch entree with just the right amount of subtle herb flavor served with nutritious Brussels sprouts.

<u>Dinner:</u> CHICKEN AND DRESSING WITH VEGETABLES

Marinated oven roasted chicken, served with a side of oriental style green beans in a ginger sauce, a walnut bread dressing, and cranberry sauce.

WEDNESDAY:

<u>Breakfast:</u> SSHE'S ORIGINAL FRUIT GRANOLA BAR

With grape juice.

<u>Lunch:</u> CHICKEN WITH PINEAPPLE SAUCE

A boneless chicken breast covered with pineapple chunks and julienne carrots in a Hawaiian sauce sprinkled with bread crumbs and baked, served with our healthy version of slaw and crunchy wheat crackers.

<u>Dinner:</u> SIGNATURE PIZZA

A generous portion of fresh tasty pizza with trendy toppings.
Served with tropical fruit salad.
This is a Seattle Sutton's kitchen specialty with universal appeal.

THURSDAY:

<u>Breakfast:</u> COUNTRY PANCAKES

With blueberry topping and grapefruit juice.

<u>Lunch:</u> SLICED CHICKEN SANDWICH

Sliced chicken on fresh baked wheat bread with tangy mustard, seasonal fruit, and crunchy chips.

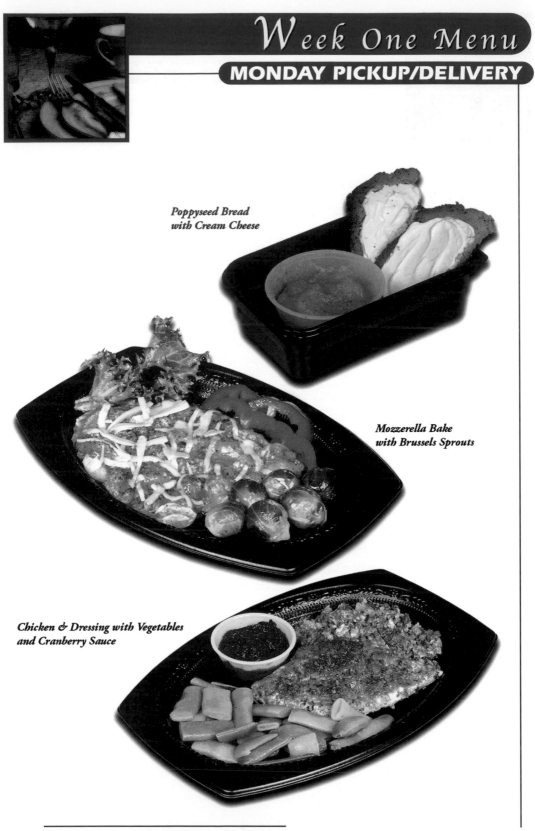

*Poppyseed Bread
with Cream Cheese*

*Mozzerella Bake
with Brussels Sprouts*

*Chicken & Dressing with Vegetables
and Cranberry Sauce*

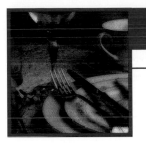

(THURSDAY:)
Dinner: TURKEY PARMESAN

Sliced breast of turkey with simply delicious basil cheese sauce served with asparagus and parsleyed potatoes.

(FRIDAY:)
Breakfast: OLD-FASHIONED BANANA BREAD

& the best fresh fruit of the season.

Lunch: PICNIC SALAD

Homemade cheese dip made from mild Cheddar and Monterey Jack cheese served with a bagel, accompanied by a toss of snow peas, red and yellow peppers and purple cabbage in a lime juice mixture.

Dinner: BAKED FISH ALMONDINE

A baked cod fillet lightly sprinkled with a Parmesan cheese topping garnished with sliced almonds, served with roasted quartered potatoes, snap peas & peach nectar.

(SATURDAY:)
Breakfast: ENGLISH MUFFIN & ROASTED PEANUT BUTTER

With select juicy bing cherries.

Lunch: CHICKEN SALAD ON MARBLE RYE

Tender morsels of white meat, fresh celery pieces and onion bits tossed in a flavorfully seasoned dressing served on hearty rye bread, accompanied by fresh fruit.

Dinner: ROSALEE'S STUFFED SHELLS

Jumbo pasta shells stuffed with Florentine and cheese in a tomato pesto sauce, served with a fresh garden salad, tasty dressing and garlic breadstick.

(SUNDAY:)
Breakfast: BLUEBERRY CHEESE BLINTZ

With breakfast juice.

Lunch: TERIYAKI CHICKEN SANDWICH

A chilled marinated chicken fillet seasoned with tarragon, chives and parsley, served with a fresh baked bun and fruit.

Dinner: RICE CONQUESTO

Homemade red beans and rice baked to perfection with a cheese topping and a side dish of stewed tomatoes, served with a delectable corn muffin.

(MONDAY:)
Breakfast: HOMEMADE GRANOLA AND FRUIT

Lunch: TURKEY LINK WORLD FAIR SPECIAL

A sausage link on a whole wheat bun topped with chili, perfect with baked potato chips.

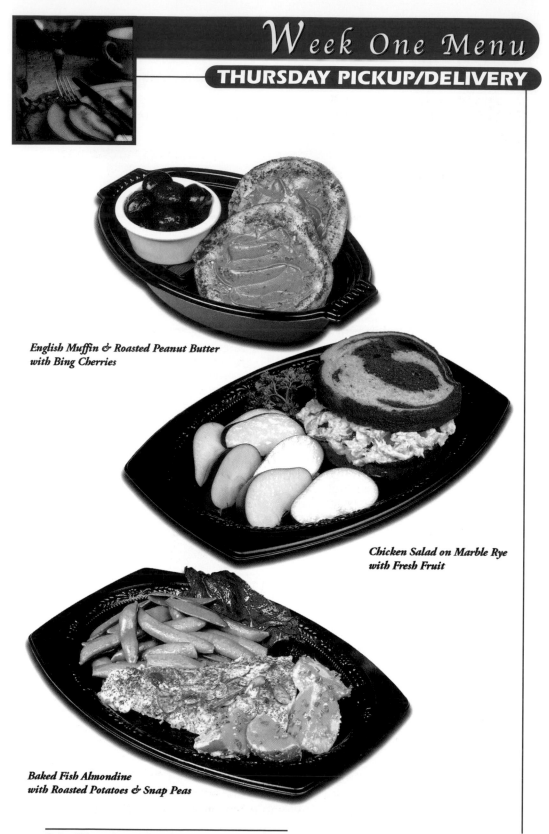

*English Muffin & Roasted Peanut Butter
with Bing Cherries*

*Chicken Salad on Marble Rye
with Fresh Fruit*

*Baked Fish Almondine
with Roasted Potatoes & Snap Peas*

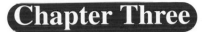

Chapter Three

In third grade, my mother gave me a little nursing kit for Christmas. It contained a stethoscope, and all kinds of neat medical stuff, so I could pretend to be a nurse. Dear Mom! Did she realize she was encouraging me to go into nursing?

That same year my dad arrived at a final conclusion that farming was not for him. He decided to move us into Gackle, and start a business.

He began by selling International Harvester equipment, and quickly expanded to become a car dealer. He was a very good salesman and a genuine community leader. People truly liked him. He knew how to treat them in a fair way, and still make money. I'm proud to be a Remboldt.

My dad loved to laugh. He had a way of friendly teasing, much of which came in the form of clever remarks. He also was fond of practical jokes, and had a glass with a hole in it. Anyone who tried to drink got soaked.

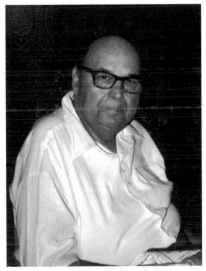

My father, Emanual Remboldt

Soon he became Mayor Remboldt, and successfully led an effort to bring paved roads and running water to Gackle. He was very active, and loved the town.

To this day, I remember him telling me that if I needed to buy something, first check it's availability in Gackle. If you can find it there, he said, buy it there. Support your community!

Of course, that's one reason Seattle Sutton's Healthy Eating is

No Gimmicks 27

headquartered in Ottawa, and employs people from Ottawa, and Marseilles, and other nearby communities. Also, the printing of this book, and the proofing, and the distribution, are contracted locally.

We purchase our International Trucks from the Ottawa dealer—men we trust—like Terry Burke at J. Merle Jones.

We could operate from anywhere now! But being in a large metropolitan area is not necessarily for the best. Here in Ottawa, we know the people with whom we do business. We trust each other. We meet each other's needs. Gladly.

My dad's advice is still on target. I'm not surprised. He was an intelligent man. Okay, I admit my bias. He was a very, very close friend of mine, and constantly did things to show me he really cared. Both my parents treated me this way. Probably that's the root of developing self-confidence in a child. I know that my parents were not formally educated on how to raise children. I think they were helped by their own upbringing.

Today's parents, even if they haven't been taught by example, have many opportunities to learn excellent ways to raise their children. Just think! If every child had a chance to feel loved and confident, wouldn't that be a better world?

I loved to play jacks, and got to be quite good. Because I usually beat all the local kids, I called myself the North Dakota champion. Jacks champion! Not a bad fantasy. My friend Monica did beat me once in a while, so my title claim was not exactly unchallengeable.

Gackle didn't have proms, or anything like that. When I was in eighth grade, though, the town had a carnival to make money for the school, and the organizers sold tickets. Each one equaled a point for a carnival queen candidate.

My father arranged with several of the sellers to come to him any time I got behind in the tally. Then he bought tickets in my name to put me in first place.

As this raised money for the school, he didn't care, and neither did the organizers, who were doing the same thing with other parents. But my dad would not be "out-bought," even though we didn't have as much money as many in town. He knew his cash was going to a good cause.

I became the carnival queen. Happy girl!

My mother's mother—Grandmother Zenker—came to America with her parents when she was 16. She was very loyal to the United States, but still had relatives living in Germany. She even wrote letters to them during World War II.

I remember D-Day, and VE-Day. Victory in Europe. Peace for everyone. I had a friend whose brother was a prisoner of the Nazis. We were very joyful about his return home.

German was my first language. Grandmother Zenker insisted that her grandchildren become fluent in German. We loved to talk with her.

Learning English was easy, when the time came.

When we are young, the human brain is primed to rapidly acquire linguistic skills—in one language, or two, or more. Concepts and objects are easily turned into verbal symbols. Sentence structure quickly follows.

Before long, my sister and I regularly communicated in English. But not in front of Grandmother Zenker.

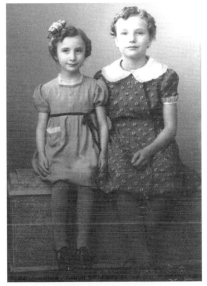

Me and Aleaine

My dad was able to finish two years of high school before he had to quit and work on the farm. My mother didn't have any educational opportunities after eighth grade, and even before then, school was a privilege, not a priority.

Not having an education didn't mean she wasn't smart. When we moved to town and Dad entered the business world, Mom did the bookkeeping.

My father was a first-rate salesman, but my mother managed the cash flow. She made sure the money worked.

I constantly learned from both of them. They wanted me to finish high school. After all, isn't it a "good parent" trait to give their beloved children new advantages? To advance generation by generation? I consider this another example of the power of love in the material world.

Of course, I also worked. On Saturdays I helped a banker, who was on the school board, handle the district's accounting. Mainly I wrote numbers in a ledger, and did the math. I also took an afternoon job as a sales clerk at the local drug store. In the evening, I sold tickets at the local theater.

It didn't really matter to me how much I got paid. Anything, I thought, is better than nothing.

When I was 13, I suddenly became very ill. I thought I should rest in bed until I felt better, but the Gackle doctor, called in by my parents, disagreed. His name was Dr. Miracle. I promise! He diagnosed my ruptured appendix and sent me forty miles to Jamestown for emergency surgery that saved my life.

I am now resisting the urge to pun his name.

My dad kept building his business portfolio, and I loved to help him. He bought a Standard Oil station and allowed me to pump fuel, which women really didn't do at that time. But I did…until the day I spilled too much gas.

Gackle High School was not large. Only fourteen people were in my graduating class. There were many opportunities for someone with energy to burn.

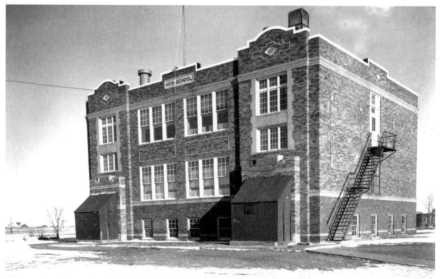

Gackle Elementary and High School

I played tenor saxophone in the band. I remember performing "O Holy Night" as a sax solo in a Christmas recital.

We weren't a good band, although we played many different

marches. The trombone players didn't know a flat from sharp. They never had a lesson, and had no music background, but were proud to be in the GHS band. So was I. We had fun together. We were friends. We were young.

I don't know how well I played, given strict evaluation standards, but I was one of the only people who could read notes (thanks to my piano lessons), and that's why I was chosen to play a solo at the Christmas concert.

We also had a pep band. I was in it, and I was a cheerleader. During a game I would run between the pep band and the cheerleader stand while my mom and dad beamed their pride.

Oh yes, I also was a majorette. Anyone could be. All it required was a willingness to practice. We made our own majorette uniforms. So fashion design went on my resume. As did my stint as editor of the school paper.

Nothing like a class of fourteen to make you look good in the yearbook. In fact, all of us were terrific. Another thing…we had no cliques or secret societies…as far as I know.

Because the school system didn't have a home economics curriculum, I joined the Gackle 4-H Club. Altogether, I belonged to 4-H for 8 years, beginning in third grade. I still treasure the award pins I received.

The local people who served as 4-H leaders were outstanding. They taught us how to cook, and sew, and freeze food. I still benefit from their influence, and I know their tradition continues to this day.

In particular, I remember a red corduroy skirt and jacket with a black silk lining I made and modeled at a 4-H fair in Jamestown. I always went for the complicated things, and maybe made a lot of errors. Not with that suit though. I'm still proud of it.

My father noted how busy I was with school and work. He established one rule: "It doesn't matter if you're up late on Saturday night as long as you make it to church on Sunday morning."

The Remboldts were Baptists, and the Zenkers were Lutheran. In those days, the wife always became associated with the religion of her husband. Though Mom was relatively new to the fold, she became a more conscientious Baptist than my dad.

He liked to have fun. For instance, he loved poker, and would arrange big games—small stakes—in the garage. That was not an acceptable Baptist practice. He also allowed me to go to movies and dances. Way back then, going to the theater and tripping the light fantastic were not condoned by some Baptists.

Those kinds of things have changed. For the better. We are meant to enjoy life, and be happy.

One of the things my mother tells me she remembers about country religion is that, if a baby died or something else bad happened, people in the church would always say, "Well, there's a reason. Or it wouldn't have happened to you." That just made it worse for the parents.

My mother said she always felt that approach was terribly unloving and cold-hearted. And I agree.

Gackle didn't have a hospital in those days. Some years after I left, a small hospital was established, but eventually it had to close and re-open as a Care Center for senior citizens. Not a nursing home. You have to go to Jamestown for that.

If a person is able to walk and use the bathroom, the strong preference is the Gackle Care Center. The food is excellent, the staff is friendly, the care is wonderful. As an added bonus, since everyone knows everyone, most visitors can spend time with every resident. It's really a social thing. Sometimes the friendships date back seventy years or longer.

When my son Chris and I visited Aunt Emma at the Gackle Care Center, he commented, "This is really nice. When can I make my reservation?"

One of my closest childhood friends was my first cousin, Maggie. To this day, we never fail to enjoy ourselves when we are together. I used to love to visit Maggie's farm and nurse the little lambs with a baby bottle.

Maggie attended a country school through 8th grade. I was really looking forward to going to high school with her. But her parents decided they needed her help on the farm.

My concern for her brought me to tears. Maybe I was just being selfish. I did want to spend more time with her.

Well, her parents had their way, and she didn't go on to school. She worked on the farm and eventually married a farmer named Leroy. They have a beautiful family, and Maggie is very happy, and always has been.

Another of my friends in high school was a girl named Annetta. We shared a fancy that we sounded good singing together. She came to my home, and we played the piano together, and sang. It may have been the kindness of the community, but we were asked to sing duets in local churches. Of course we accepted.

To this day, when I think of Annetta (now called Anne), I think of singing. I see her every time I go back to Gackle, because she's the local hairdresser, and a member of the Baptist Church. Her face always makes me smile.

Barn dances were popular during the years when I was in high school, or home from college. In the Gackle area, these gatherings were a rite of fall, held at the conclusion of the harvest. A year of hard work had coaxed life-giving treasure from the soil, and now a grateful population paused to celebrate.

Barn dances were also called sunrise dances, because they continued until the sun came up. I'm glad I convinced my dad that nobody ever died from lack of sleep.

We danced all night—usually to the music of a single accordion in the hayloft. Everyone had energy to burn. We never drank alcohol. We never even thought about drinking it.

We girls preferred to go to a sunrise dance without dates. We did not want to be there with a boyfriend, because, then, we couldn't dance with all the other boys.

Since my dad was in the automobile business, I always had access to some kind of used car and could drive my friends. We did not allow the boys to ride with us.

Oh, how I love to welcome the sunrise after a night of dancing. The whole experience was such total fun. Nothing topped it.

Nowadays, when I look back at Gackle and think of my friends, time becomes irrelevant. Every memory seems to reference something that might have happened at dawn today, or yesterday evening at the latest. We genuinely liked and cared for each other. Yes, friendship is stronger than time.

Well it was wonderful, but I don't want to mislead. It wasn't paradise. We had our disagreements. We worked through our differences, because it was a small town, and we didn't have a choice.

Good. I'm glad. Getting past the unimportant squabbles sweetened our friendships. Learning to accommodate the concerns of others strengthened them.

If you like someone, you can be assured that they will like you too. Not always true? Eventually it is, or so I believe, once two people get to know each other.

Speaking of time, my life in Gackle seemed to last an eternity. Seattle Sutton's Theory of Relativity: a year lasted longer when I was younger. Now each one passes so quickly. Perspective, I guess.

When you are a child, and it's the last afternoon of the last day of class, and Memorial Day isn't until next Monday, the 90-plus days until school starts again seem like forever. How long does the same time period feel when you're an adult?

When I assess the influence of my parents on my career, I think it is obvious that my entrepreneurship came from my father. My mother, on the other hand, always wanted to be a nurse, but never had the opportunity. Her frustrated desire, and my respect and love for her, definitely had a strong impact on my decision to go into nursing.

My parents did not put pressure on me to go to college. They liked the idea, but knew I could be happy in Gackle. And we would have enjoyed living in proximity.

One of my relatives (on my father's side), however, was a principal at the high school, and another was a businessman.

They each talked with me about the brand new nursing program at Jamestown College, forty miles away. I soon realized I could go there for four years and three summers and receive my R. N. and a Bachelor of Science degree. I believe there were only eleven such nursing programs in the nation in 1950.

Please permit me a short digression. I must mention that our nation is facing a nursing crisis. Within a few years, we're going to be short almost 800,000 nurses. If the problem is not solved, some intensive care units will be forced to close.

If you like to work hard and help people, perhaps you should be a nurse. Maybe you'll have the same anticipatory feeling I did in the summer of 1950, when I decided to enroll in Jamestown College.

My parents supported my decision, though they realized if I went that route, I would never live in Gackle again. I knew it too. And it troubled me.

But never to live in Gackle again is not the same as never visiting Gackle again. Vowing to return many times (a promise I have gladly kept), I made peace with my choice, and in 1950 left for Jamestown College.

Once I arrived and started school, I received an unexpected Gackle bonus. Jamestown had a hospital, and the college's nurses-in-training were associated with it. Many people from Gackle were admitted there, and more than a few couldn't speak English.

I was called upon many times to translate—German to English & vice versa—for patients and medical staff. Thanks, Grandmother Zenker.

It made me proud because I was helping patients who knew my parents and me. Everyone knows everyone in a town of 500 people.

Translating to assist the healing process jump-started my nursing career. Something basic in me responded to the observable positives I was putting in the mix. I felt more alive than ever…and I always feel very much alive.

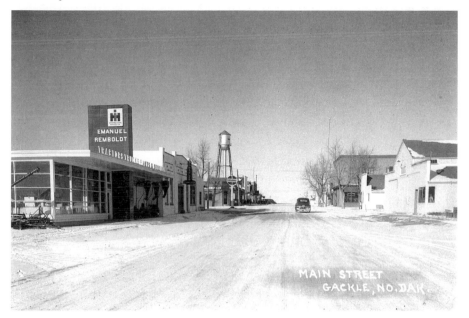

Dad's implement business is on the left

Helping people is a primary human motivation, at least for me. The web of life…and all that. In those moments of translation, I knew, with a heart-soaring clarity, that, without a doubt, nursing—and Jamestown College School of Nursing—had been excellent choices.

Chapter Four

My primary family concern while at Jamestown was my dad's health. He and I had been very close all my life, particularly in high school. We both loved to talk, especially with each other.

Dad kept gaining weight, though, and by the time I left for college, he had reached 385 pounds. Eventually he had to be hospitalized. The doctors cautioned him to lose one hundred pounds or face the prospect of congestive heart failure, like his parents, and other relatives. "Emanuel," the doctors said, "lose or die."

The situation frightened my mother. Of course, she desired with all her heart for Dad to live, but at the same time she wanted to please him. He always insisted on eating the foods he liked in the quantities he considered sufficient to appease his hunger. Limiting him was difficult, since our meals were served family style—which meant large portions and second helpings. Many people who survived the depression shared a common thought: "Don't run out of food."

Mom prepared many delicious German dishes. She was a remarkably good cook. Her homemade noodles and strudels could not be topped, even after she no longer traveled to the mill to grind the wheat.

She tried hard to cook healthy food for Dad, and to serve smaller portions to help him lose weight. He struggled valiantly to comply, enjoyed a little success, and then backslid, just like almost everyone does.

My Mother knew my Dad was eating too much. What could she do? He wanted to eat the way he wanted to eat.

I thought, "If someone knew how to make calorie-controlled meals, he would have results, and therefore gain confidence. After all, his only alternative is an early death from congestive heart failure."

That's why I kept sending menu plans.

Meanwhile, I continued my education at Jamestown College, where my unusual first name unexpectedly proved to be an asset. People remembered "Seattle." I think that's why I was elected to be a cheerleader for the Jamestown Jimmies football team.

We fledgling nurses learned basic nutrition as part of our curriculum. The bottom line never changes: calorie intake versus calorie output. People conjure an endless chain of superficially logical gimmicks, but losing weight always comes down to one simple fact.

Burn more calories than you consume, and lose; burn less, and gain.

We did most of our clinical training at Jamestown Hospital, near the college. J. H. only had 90 beds. As our education progressed, we eventually mastered the challenges and routines of a small hospital. We received our caps in 1951.

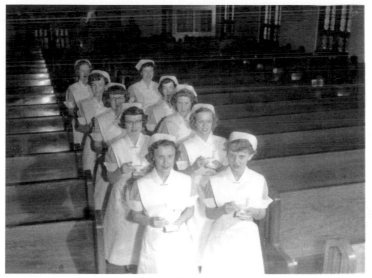

I'm the front nurse on the left during our capping ceremony

At a certain point in their education, determined by the college administrators, its nurses-in-training were sent to learn while affiliating with larger hospitals for nine months.

My group's first assignment was Cook County Hospital in Chicago. That busy and frantic atmosphere was quite an experience—especially for a girl who grew up in Gackle.

All nine of us were apprehensive as we stepped from the Jamestown platform onto the train. To tell the truth, we were afraid. The trip—maybe just the idea of living in a totally urban environment—made our heads spin.

Iron wheels relentlessly click-clacked on steel tracks, separating us from home, minute by minute, mile by mile. All the while, we stared out at the passing vistas, framed like a movie by railroad car windows, each scene rushing into view and just as quickly disappearing. The effect was hypnotic, lulling us into a warm anticipatory cocoon. We were on our way to the Big City! Wow!

Finally the locomotive pulled us into the station. The motion of the wheels—and scenery—halted. The security and safety of our small town life melted away as we departed the train and began a cautious trek through unprecedented (for us) traffic, noise, and masses of people.

Like millions before and since, we made a successful transition from rural to urban life. Our small town hospital experience turned out to be a huge plus. In many ways, we were more versatile than the other nurses-in-training, having been taught how to draw blood, start IVs, and carry out hospital basics.

Our confidence quickly grew as we realized we could do more than Cook County required of us. The big city hospital had residents and interns to carry out many tasks that had been our routine duties at Jamestown.

Rather than being behind, as we had feared, we were actually ahead. Which didn't make us less busy. Nurses historically are overworked.

Some people think that, when it comes to relating to patients, nurses are personal, and doctors are impersonal. My experience is that some doctors are personal and some aren't. Often you can't tell from a few hospital interactions, because sometimes the doctor may be rushing from patient to patient. A nurse spends more time with each one.

I preferred to work directly with the sick. The administrative side didn't interest me, although it may be much easier. In my experience very few nurses chose the administrative over the "hands-on."

Back in 1952, at Cook County, all nurses-in-training rotated through several "specialty" areas. My first assignment was "Contagion." This was the height of the polio epidemic. I remember large rooms filled with respirators.

A dentist and his wife, both suffering from polio, were in separate respirators. I took care of them—feeding, bathing, everything. They could do nothing for themselves.

And they were by no means the only ones. Polio was a ravaging disease. To watch it attack its victims was heart wrenching.

The vaccine changed everything. I am so grateful for Jonas Salk.

Not to be flip, but I am also filled head-to-toe with sincere gratitude for one of my classmates. She was dating a guy who had a friend, you know how that goes.

The friend's name was Kelly, a pleasant fellow who earned his undergraduate degree from the University of Illinois in Urbana, and his medical credentials from the University of Illinois Medical School in Chicago.

It wasn't long before our friends tried to arrange a "fix-up." I said, "Sure, I'll go." He also answered in the affirmative.

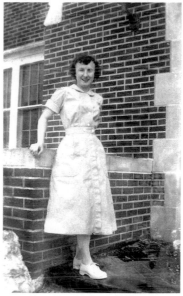
Ah, the waist of youth

At first, I didn't know what to think about this man. His character was hard to gauge. Was he nice? Or not? He certainly didn't gush over me. He seemed too quiet…and yet completely natural. And what about his peculiar sense of humor?

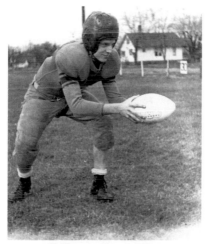
Kelly on the gridiron

The more I came to know him, the more I realized how much I liked him. He wasn't phony like some of the guys I had dated. He had an honest and forthright manner. I could tell he wasn't just getting to know any woman, he was getting to know me.

Our courtship in Chicago was brief. My class, having completed six months of training in Chicago, divided into two groups. Four of us were sent to Pueblo, Colorado, for three months of psychiatric training.

The location couldn't have been lovelier, and the hospital was as beautiful as the scenery. Many of the patients were alcoholics. A normal detoxification took nine months. Other patients stayed varying terms. Some were never discharged.

The hospital had its own farm, partially maintained and worked by the patients. The specialty of the farm's garden was raspberries. Very tasty. Healthy eating!

We trained and worked from 6 a.m. to 2 p.m., taking our meals in the cafeteria. Oh my gosh, the food was great.

It struck me that most of the patients were able to function well enough, even though they were, for all practical purposes, prisoners.

They not only helped on the farm, but in the hospital, and the cafeteria. Work seemed a plus in their lives…something central and real to help them organize their thoughts and structure their day.

Kelly and I kept in contact via letters. Not frequently, though. I was dating other guys, and I supposed he was doing the same, except with women.

My summer was excellent. Finishing work at 2 p.m. gave us the afternoon and early evening to play. We found a place to swim with a thrilling diving cliff, and went there almost every day. I even bought a ukulele and learned to play.

I never phoned Kelly and he never called me. In that era, long distance calls just weren't made for such purposes. Too expensive.

Three months passed quickly. Soon it was time to head back to Jamestown. By then, we were ready to go home.

We traveled by bus from Pueblo to Omaha, Nebraska. We had reservations from Omaha to Breckenridge, Minnesota, home of my college roommate, and, from there, to Jamestown.

It was quite a trip, but as can happen with transportation in any era, whether stagecoaches in the old west, or jet planes in the modern world, things don't always go as planned. Our initial leg was slowed by a bad storm. By the time we pulled into Omaha, the bus for Breckinridge had already departed.

Four young women stranded in a strange city! We had our tickets, and a box of Ritz Crackers (portion control!), but that was about all. We checked the airport for flights out. Nothing scheduled all weekend.

What could we do? Well, we weren't completely bereft of resources. We had confidence. We had courage.

So we tried something that might not be wise in the 21st century. Wearing Jamestown College jackets, we took up positions by the side of the road, thumbs up and out. With a crayon, I scrawled "On To Minnesota" on my white ukulele carrying case, and held it high for drivers to see.

We made a basic decision that we would not separate. If a potential ride only had room for one of us, that would not do. All or none!

The first driver to stop was a game warden. We rode with him for quite a while. Then, just as it was beginning to get dark, he stopped and told us, "I am going to leave you here, but I live right down the road." He pointed. "If you don't get another ride, walk to my house, and my wife and I will put you up for the night."

Well, it wasn't but a minute or so, and another vehicle stopped. A furniture truck. We rode in the back.

When that ride was over, we didn't have to wait very long for a third. An elderly couple. We piled into the back seat, and sang to entertain them. I remember playing two songs on my ukulele: "You Are My Sunshine," and "Goodnight, Irene."

Our last ride was with a fellow who truly enjoyed high speed driving. As the car flew through the night, we studied the bus schedule, and suddenly realized we had made such good time hitching that we had a chance to catch up with our bus in Breckenridge.

Our driver accepted the challenge and increased his already rapid pace. I'm not kidding. He drove really, really, really fast! This in a time of no seat belts.

Ralph Waldo Emerson: "I never rode in a coach that went fast enough for me." Well, he "never rode" with this guy!

We braced on whatever part of the car we could grasp, and scrutinized oncoming traffic with wide eyes and rapidly beating hearts. I guess everyone has had times when accepting a challenge resulted in the assumption of unusual (and unnecessary) risk, and something bad might have happened, but didn't.

Our speed racer delivered us to the depot just in time. We caught up with the bus we had missed! We shorted ourselves a leg of the journey, but had an adventure.

The four of us clambered on board, took our seats, sighed deeply, looked at each other, and grinned in unfeigned sisterhood.

Of course, we informed our parents—many years later. I also told the story to my daughter, Paula when I gave her that same ukulele.

The episode did inspire me with an entrepreneurial thought. What about a system matching hitchhikers with drivers? Background checks for all involved. Special identifying cards. Cars filled with strangers getting to know each other, and beginning new friendships.

I spent a few days mulling the concept. But cards can be stolen…and the liability…too much. Sometimes the best thing about having an exciting idea is knowing when to drop it.

Fortified by three years of on-the-job training and education, I began my senior year at Jamestown College. I respect the hard-working people who earn their R.N. degree at a hospital, but the experience of combining a nursing and general college atmosphere helped round out my education. Part of my curriculum included such classes as music appreciation, literature, religion, and philosophy. Plus, at a college, there are boys!

Which brings me back to Kelly. Our letters continued and got more… interesting. When Kelly's classmate—the one dating mine—decided to come for a visit, the prospect very much excited my friend and caused me to pause, gaze at the stars, and wonder.

Not for long. Kelly wrote and asked if I would mind if he came to see me. No, I wouldn't!

He and his friend answered an ad in the Chicago Tribune seeking someone to deliver a pick-up truck to North Dakota. They were selected for the job, and given twenty dollars for gas.

They each sold a pint of blood and used the money to purchase a train ticket from Jamestown to Chicago. Then, taking turns driving, they gobbled up the miles between Chicago and Fargo, where they dropped off the truck, and hitchhiked a hundred miles to Jamestown to visit us for the weekend.

My roommate had an aunt and uncle in Jamestown. The boys stayed there. We had a very good time. The girls and the boys, I mean. I couldn't say what kind of time the aunt and uncle had.

More Relativity Theory: Friday, Saturday, and Sunday didn't last as long as three normal days. It seemed only a couple of hours before it was time for our two visitors to board the train and head back to the University of Illinois Medical School in Chicago.

As you know, I was familiar with the railroad voyage from Jamestown to Chicago, and I could imagine every click-clack of his ride home. By the way, that route—so important in my life—no longer exists. Isn't that the way it goes?

Before Kelly heeded the "All Aboard," he handed me his fraternity pin. "What does this mean?" I asked. His answer: "Just that somebody from Illinois cares about you."

How like him not to put any pressure on me! Didn't ask me not to date others. Didn't tell me he wasn't dating anyone else. What a guy!

We continued to write. Then, in the winter of 1954, with my state boards coming up in June, I visited him in Chicago. That's when he proposed. "Let's get married." As straight forward as that. I said yes, with a caveat. Before we planned the wedding, I wanted to study for my state boards, and get that out of the way first. He understood completely.

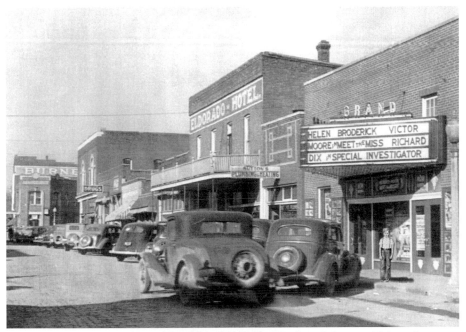

You can see Kelly in the right foreground of main street Eldorado

Then Kelly informed me that his parents and relatives in southern Illinois hadn't heard a word about our dating—didn't know that I existed, let alone that he had proposed. Here's how he told them: "I'm getting married to Seattle from Gackle." They still tease me about the parsimony of his initial description.

I studied for my boards all right. But I also found time to design and sew my own wedding trousseau: a satin dress with a long train and a lace top. I sewed the gauntlets too, and the veil. The beaded crown came from my mother's wedding.

An engagement ring might have been nice, but given our financial situation, it seemed an unwise extravagance. He had no extra money to buy one, and thought it foolish to borrow. So did I. Why should we pay interest for something we didn't need?

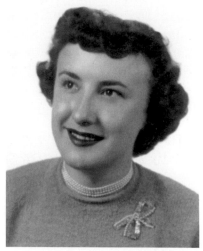

This is the picture my parents used to announce our engagement

Our wedding rings were ordered from a Montgomery Ward catalogue. They cost $13.98 apiece (as I remember), and were shipped C.O.D. When they arrived, we learned we had been the beneficiary of a sale, and the price had been lowered to nine dollars and a few cents each.

We were wed on Aug. 23, 1954. Closing in on fifty years.

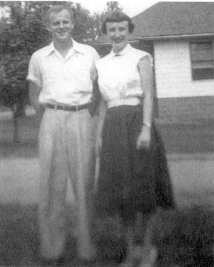

The happy newlyweds

Those mail order rings worked out just fine. Still as good as new.

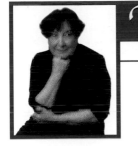

Have compassion for the overweight child, because such a condition reaches into the future, affecting self-esteem, health, education, marriage, and employment. Overweight children tend to become overweight adults.

When a child is obese, the parent has the responsibility to help by making sure only the right (healthy) foods are available and served in sensible portions.

Parents need to encourage any interest in sports, whether it be volleyball, swimming, basketball, bicycling, skateboarding, bowling, or whatever. If nothing else is available, four or five times a week, walk a couple of miles with your child.

Simply put: Responsible parents absolutely must do everything within their power to make sure that their children are not overweight. Use your thinking rights.

The process begins with pregnancy. Mothers need to eat healthy. No fad diets. Limit fast foods and junk foods. This is as important as no smoking, no alcohol, and no drugs. A baby in the womb is a prisoner of its mother's diet.

It's also important not to gain too much weight. Sometimes women in pregnancy must deal with powerful urges to eat particular foods. Possibly pickles. Or ice cream. If it's ice cream, control it. Remember, you really aren't eating calories for two.

I believe all infants deserve to be breastfed. This benefits the child and the mother, because the latest studies I have read indicate breastfeeding reduces the odds of breast malignancies for a lifetime. Being breastfed also reduces the child's risk of breast cancer later in life.

The breastfeeding mother—for her sake, and that of her child—should use extra caution and extra willpower to stay on a balanced, healthy, diet.

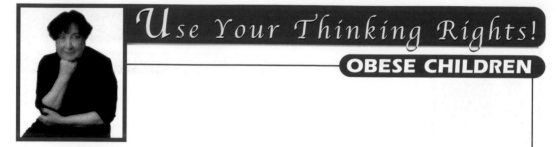

Use Your Thinking Rights!

OBESE CHILDREN

Mothers have a tendency to stop a toddler from crying by offering candy or a cookie. Behaviorally speaking, this is a counter-productive conditioner. The acquired response is: "I can eat when I'm not hungry."

We live in the horn of plenty. Food is more abundant here and now than any other time and any other place. The most asked question in our society, wherever we go, is, "Are you hungry?"

With such an emphasis on food, overeating is likely, even inevitable, especially if the answer to the above question is an unthinking "yes" rather than a truthful "no." Extra calories quickly turn into extra pounds.

The World Health Organization reports: "The fundamental causes of the obesity epidemic are sedentary lifestyles and high-fat, energy-dense diets."

Let me paraphrase this as it applies to children: "Too much TV and video games, too much junk and fast food."

Parents need to use their thinking rights to guard their children's health.

As overweight children become overweight adults, diseases associated with excess poundage are likely to become more frequent and more immediate.

Equally disturbing, more children are being diagnosed with obesity-related diseases that doctors once saw almost exclusively in overweight adults.

Parents, if your child is overweight, make no excuse. The need for action is known. The importance cannot be denied. The consequences are dire.

Yet the solution is available. Eat right. Exercise more.

For most children, this will do the trick.

The very few who may have other circumstances affecting their weight will need medical assistance.

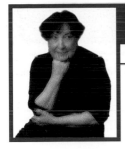

I now position my fingers on the keyboard to express my support for a tasty and pleasing food with an unfairly sullied reputation. I write of that eminently satisfactory fly-catcher, sugar, whose nutritional reputation science has finally restored.

Sugar is a form of carbohydrate, and carbohydrates are an excellent source of energy. One teaspoon of sugar has 40% fewer calories than an equal serving of fat.

Many years ago people thought that sugar caused children to be hyperactive. But scientific studies have proven this is not true. Sugar is not a cause of hyperactivity. It is an energy food that can stimulate activity.

Numerous scientific studies have confirmed that consumption of sugar does not cause chronic diseases such as obesity, diabetes, heart disease, hyperactivity, nor does it contribute to deficiency in the diet by displacing other more valuable nutrients. There is no reason to avoid table sugar in favor of other sweeteners, especially those mysterious artificial concoctions.

For most of the past one hundred years, people with diabetes were told to avoid sugar. It was assumed that sugar, which quickly changes into glucose, would raise blood glucose levels significantly more than other foods. But research has shown this is not true. For example, the glycemic index, which measures how much a specific food is likely to increase your blood sugar, is actually higher for split pea soup than for table sugar.

All digestible complex dietary carbohydrates are broken down to simple sugars in the stomach and intestines before they are absorbed into the body.

On the flip side, sugar foods are often empty calories.

Use your thinking rights. Sugar is just fine in moderation, but it should not replace other carbohydrates that supply vitamins and minerals.

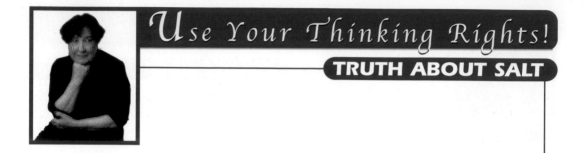

I find it kind of odd when people tell me they need a salt/sodium free diet.

People die if they don't eat salt. So a complete prohibition is a death warrant. That's why cows need to lick salt blocks.

Of course there's enough sodium in prepared foods that even people who never reach for a salt shaker get more than enough. Most people probably take in twice as much salt as they really need.

A growing number of reports suggest that salt intake risks have been exaggerated. True, too much salt raises the blood pressure of some people, but for others it doesn't. If you are one of the former, your diet needs to be sodium- restricted. On the other hand, salt usually poses no threat to people with normal kidneys and normal blood pressure.

Moderation is more than a virtue, it's wisdom.

But it is neither wise nor necessary to fear a modicum of salt falling from its shaker onto your food.

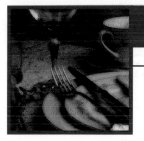

MONDAY:

Dinner: CHICKEN & LINGUINI

Baked chicken rolled in Parmesan cheese on linguini topped with tomato sauce and a side of herb enhanced zucchini slices.

TUESDAY:

Breakfast: LUSCIOUS STRAWBERRY BREAD

With citrus sections.

Lunch: TENDER TURKEY FILLET SANDWICH

Oven roasted turkey fillet served on a bagel with a sandwich spread and this season's fresh fruit.

Dinner: BAKED TUNA & NOODLES

A flavorful tuna casserole, chilled vinaigrette style cucumber salad and trendy petite carrots, served with a dark rye dinner roll.

WEDNESDAY:

Breakfast: MOIST AND DELICIOUS BANANA MUFFIN W/ CREAM CHEESE

With seasonal fruit.

Lunch: GAZPACHO AND CARROTS WITH SPINACH DIP

Baby carrots along with a tasty spinach dip, accompanied by a hearty gazpacho cold soup and a rye bun.

Dinner: MEATBALLS WITH POTATOES AND PEAS

Seasoned meatballs smothered in a low-fat sauce, served with potatoes au gratin and seasoned peas, an old family favorite meal.

THURSDAY:

Breakfast: RAISIN BAGEL

With cream cheese, healthy stewed dried plums, and juice.

Lunch: ECLECTIC BISTRO SANDWICH

Build your own vegetarian sandwich using Provolone cheese, slices of Roma tomato, and top with a vegetable spread. Served with fresh fruit.

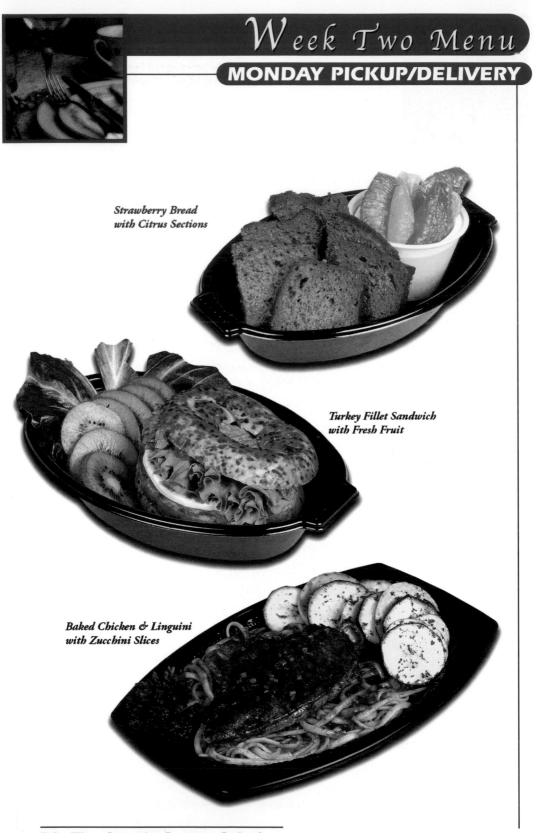

*Strawberry Bread
with Citrus Sections*

*Turkey Fillet Sandwich
with Fresh Fruit*

*Baked Chicken & Linguini
with Zucchini Slices*

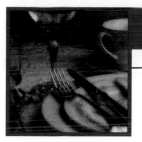

(THURSDAY:)
Dinner: SEASONED CHICKEN & POLENTA

Fillet of tender baked chicken and a vegetable combination served with Seattle Sutton's signature old-fashioned polenta Napoleon.

(FRIDAY:)
Breakfast: SENSATIONAL PUMPKIN BREAD

With raspberry yogurt.

Lunch: MANY BEAN SALAD

An assortment of fiber-rich beans in a vinaigrette dressing, served with Colby cheese, an onion bagel and fresh seasonal fruit.

Dinner: STUFFED POTATO

The trendy popular overstuffed potato with pieces of broccoli smothered with three cheeses, served with a side of slow cooked Lima beans.

(SATURDAY:)
Breakfast: WAFFLES WITH STRAWBERRY SAUCE

Lunch: VEGETARIAN SOUP AND TUNA SALAD SANDWICH

A well-seasoned vegetarian soup simmered to perfection and served with tuna salad on a fresh wheat bun.

Dinner: FAJITA MEXICANA

Fashionable chicken strips and vegetables wrapped in a tortilla shell with high-fiber refried beans, and guacamole.

(SUNDAY:)
Breakfast: OPEN FACE BREAKFAST SANDWICH

Served with juice.

Lunch: LASAGNA ROLL-UP

Pasta roll topped with a luscious mild sauce, accompanied by Paula's perfect salad combo of broccoli, cauliflower and sunflower seeds.

Dinner: CHICKEN & SWISS CHEESE CASSEROLE

A perfectly baked combination of broccoli flowerettes, tender meat, baby Swiss cheese and rice served with golden corn on the cob.

(MONDAY:)
Breakfast: SSHE'S SPECIAL BLUEBERRY MUFFIN

with Citrus Fruit

Lunch: CHICKEN SALAD SANDWICH

Tender pieces of chicken, onion bits and celery slices tossed in a creamy dressing, on a fresh baked bun. Served with fresh fruit.

No Gimmicks 51

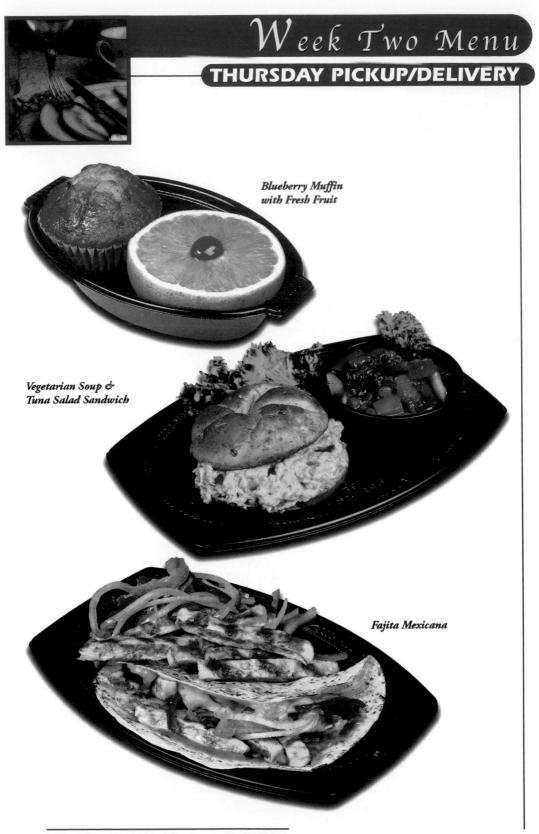

Blueberry Muffin with Fresh Fruit

Vegetarian Soup & Tuna Salad Sandwich

Fajita Mexicana

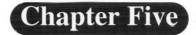
Married in August, a month after Kelly started his internship in Peoria, Illinois, at St. Francis Hospital. He was one of the first doctors to intern at St. Francis, and found it so worthwhile that he influenced ten of his friends to join him.

The St. Francis Eleven and their spouses coalesced into an instant tribe. We spent much of our time together, never lacking for entertainment, like good neighbors in a small town.

We were a natural support group. Interns work long and odd hours. Daily life would have been more difficult without our friends.

On June 26, 1955, Kelly and I had a son, Christopher. He was a breech delivery, so the birth was difficult, more so because the procedure was normal. In the present day, when a mother is having her first baby, and it is a breech, caesareans are a standard medical practice. This was not true in 1955.

No matter. I was a mother! Kelly was a father! We were a family!

If you watch too much TV, you might think stories that start this way usually end badly. I am saddened that many do.

But not ours. It never occurred to us that we weren't going to live happily ever after. And we were right! A clear demonstration that belief anticipates experience.

After he completed his internship, Kelly went into the Air Force to serve his two-year military obligation. He was assigned to McConnell AFB (home of the B-47s) in Wichita, Kansas, where we lived for two years. We did not find life in the military to be unpleasant. To the contrary, we felt the work was important, and we enjoyed the company of bright and dedicated people our own age. Not to sound like a broken record, but we had a wonderful time!

We danced a lot. Jitterbugging. And the Lindy. Don't laugh. That was my generation's way of rocking and rolling. It may seem tame now, but that's not a bad thing. When we were young, it was the cat's pajamas, if you know what I mean.

Dancing is one of the happiest human activities. Dance combines the exuberance of individual self-expression with the satisfactions of participating in a community embraced form. Moving to music is a passion we all share.

We love to dance: campfire, waltz, ball-room, jitterbug, funky chicken, ballet, or pogo. Understand the dance protocol of a culture—or a generation—and know their hearts.

Kelly didn't jitterbug that much, but he loved to go to parties. He'd dance with all the women. Years ago, we were always the last ones to leave the party.

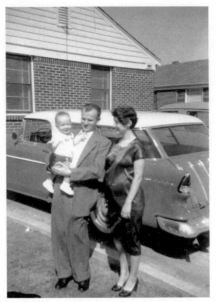

One baby in our arms, another on the way

During our stay in Kansas, I had a second baby. Paula was born in May of 1956 (ten and a half months after Chris). Kelly and I had established a goal of a dozen! We were well on our way.

Once, on leave, we went to a Lions Club near my husband's hometown of Eldorado, Illinois. We played Bingo and I won the last game's grand prize—filling the entire card. When my last number was called, I shouted: "BINGO," and checked to see if anyone else was going to share the victory. No!

The prize money went to buy a sewing machine and drapery material. Over the next several years, I made five sports coats for Kelly. I always worried about him going to someone's home wearing his coat…and maybe they would have the same fabric in their drapes.

My mother-in-law, Helen, and my father-in-law, Herman, were two of the best people in the world. I knew from the first day we met that I would always be very good to them. They were wonderful to me.

We always had a lot of laughs, and my mother-in-law became one of my best friends. Kelly and I used to visit them every summer. Three hundred miles each way. Five little children in the car.

We usually stayed for about a week. That had to be hectic for them, but I never heard a complaint.

Always, when we left, Helen stood next to our station wagon and cried. Her tears streamed down her cheeks. I couldn't help but think, "It's wonderful she hates for us to leave."

Of course, Helen and Herman often visited our house. They were always welcome. One day years later we were sitting around the table with the children, talking and talking—a real festival of gab.

The subject of her crying at our departures came up. She chuckled for a moment, and said, "That's because I was so glad to see you leave." The entire room erupted in laughter.

I don't remember any time that Kelly's parents criticized the way we raised our children. They could have. Anyone can be critical of other people. You can find an imperfection every day in everyone you know, if you want.

Or you can try to find good things and celebrate what's right. That's what Helen and Herman did.

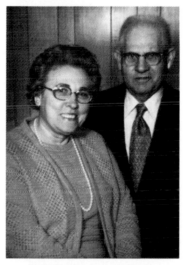

**Kelly's Mom and Dad,
Helen and Herman Sutton**

As Kelly's obligatory military service drew to a close, we gave serious consideration to staying in the Air Force. Perhaps our decision might have been different if Kelly hadn't received a call from his former classmate, Dr. Bill Hays.

Dr. Hays had fulfilled his military duty prior to attending medical school, and after his internship had immediately gone to work in a small town. He had enjoyed his experience, but now wanted to move on and take a residency in internal medicine.

His departure would leave the Illinois village of Marseilles with a doctor shortage, so he asked Kelly to take over his practice.

Kelly respected Bill, and decided to check out the offer. He traveled to Marseilles, where he was courted by the whole town. It was like a scene out of Doc Hollywood. "Come to Marseilles, Dr. Sutton. Get off the interstate. Come to Marseilles."

The town's resident medical practitioner was Dr. Paul R. Clark, who embraced Kelly like a son. Dr. Clark had earned a national reputation as a physician because of his skill in separating conjoined twins.

Paul and his friends showed Kelly the town, and the hospital in nearby Ottawa, and played many rounds of golf and many hands of poker with him. Their courtship worked.

Kelly, having grown up in a small Illinois town, liked the look and feel of this similar environment. He sought my advice and consent. What did I think?

With two children, and the prospect of more, I thought I was too busy to think. Wherever Kelly wanted to practice medicine was all right with me.

We moved to Marseilles in the fall of 1957. We rented a nice house. Not too big. In fact, it quickly became too small. Peter was born in October and now our family had three in diapers! And not disposable!

When the children were small, they needed a lot of clothing. I've never been one who cared to impress people by wearing new clothes all the time. That trait came in handy!

I even stopped purchasing new underwear for a while, figuring the tatter and tear on the old ones didn't show, and we could get something for the kids instead. Many financially conscious mothers have made like sacrifices—and more—while raising their children.

Kelly worked his practice, and I was the primary care giver for a trio of small children. We liked the town, and I guess the town liked us.

We were especially fond of the dozen or so Italian grocery stores in Marseilles. Perhaps it would be more apt to call them "sausage" stores, because most of the proprietors made their own Italian sausage.

If a house call brought him into one of these homes, Dr. Sutton would be offered ravioli, and sausage, and homemade wine. He often accepted, after his work was done, of course.

It wasn't unusual for the people Kelly treated to bring him gifts. Farmers brought us their produce—corn, tomatoes, beans, etc. They weren't doing this on a barter basis. They paid their bills. This was extra.

Dr. Clark urged Kelly to buy the house immediately east of his. Kelly was paid $1,000 a month, so the price was a little steep for a young family. To encourage us to settle in Marseilles, Dr. Clark helped with the down payment, and the realtor refused to take a commission. We closed the deal in the fall of 1958, and have lived in the same house ever since.

I had a miscarriage in 1958, and then in '59 our daughter Ruth was born. Sarah, our youngest, came in 1962.

Kelly and I decided that aiming for a dozen had been a little ambitious. We liked our children so much that we decided five would suffice.

The Sixties may have been a decade of turmoil and change, but I was busy being a mother, and much of it whizzed past my notice. Of course, like most young mothers, I wanted to communicate more with the outside world. As much as I loved my children, I didn't want them to be the boundaries of my universe. No matter how hard you try, though, for all practical purposes, until a certain age, they are.

When they were quite small, on cold weather days I used to harass them to put on hats and mittens and coats. I worried that if they didn't wear warm clothes they might catch colds.

One night at dinner, Kelly told me that "you don't catch a cold by getting cold." Hearing this, the children asked to prove his point. Kelly agreed, and, after a few minutes discussion, I reluctantly went along.

Though there was snow on the ground the following day, the kids played outside without coats, hats, gloves, or….shoes. They ran around just to prove to me that, hey, we're all getting cold, and now we'll wait and see.

"If we're not sick within two or three weeks, Mom, you'll know you don't have to tell us to put on our coats."

Well, they remained perfectly healthy. So I just never bothered or worried about that again. Not that the book was closed on the subject.

When Ruth was taking a health class in high school, the same question came up for discussion. She raised her hands and made the point that exposure to cold doesn't lead to colds. Her teacher strongly disagreed. Ruth wouldn't give in. The teacher made her sit in the hall.

Actually, Ruth was quite opinionated, and frequently suffered an identical exile. In this way, she and the school custodian, Dick Allen, became very good friends.

In 1963, our family adopted a dog. We named her Cleopatra. She was a proud mongrel, who gave us 12 litters of pups—52 in all. Her cycle—heat, pregnancy, delivery—provided a useful sex education for our children.

But placing her puppies in good homes was a challenge. Kelly finally decided to take out ads in the local paper: "Puppies For Sale. Worth $100. Will Sacrifice for 5 Cents."

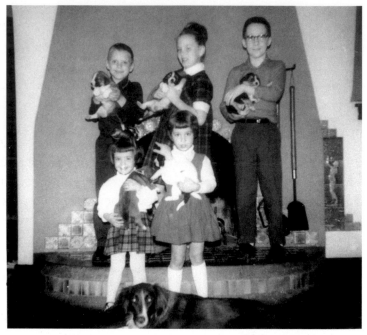

Cleo's Goal: Ten Puppies For Every Child

Cleo used to follow our children to the movies. She would sit outside and wait to lead them home. She also escorted Sarah to school. Then the dog would return to our house, and spend the day in her usual pursuits, including visiting the neighbors. But she seemed to be able to tell time, because she would always find her way back to the school to meet Sarah and walk her home. Her chronological expertise reminded me of my first dog, Mopes. Cleo lived with us for 13 years.

In November of 1963 the children had come home—from play and school—for lunch. They finished eating, and went downstairs to watch TV in the basement and enjoy the antics of Bozo the Clown. Kelly and I were eating lunch together upstairs.

A clatter on the stairs preceded terrible news.

Chris shouted: "The president has been assassinated."

We turned on the upstairs TV and radio. Almost immediately the news was confirmed. Horrible! Horrible! For his family. For the people. For the country. Absolutely horrible.

We thought Kennedy was a great President. Everyone I knew—Republican and Democrat—was really upset. In retrospect, I can see that this was a turning point, allowing sadness and mistrust a disproportionate presence in the collective American psyche. I don't know if we're over it yet.

It would help if we knew for certain what happened to JFK. Even that probably wouldn't be enough. We really need another president like him. But that doesn't happen very often. That's why he was special.

Even though he wasn't a United States president, I felt just as sad when Martin Luther King was killed. He was courageous and articulate, and helped put the country on the right path.

I don't consider myself a prejudiced person. Everyone is more comfortable with what they know best—their familiar surroundings and cultural frame of reference. That's not prejudice. That's natural.

The point is to be aware that, underneath the differences, we're all human, and, therefore, fundamentally linked. This is so simple, and so often said, and yet needs to be repeated, and absorbed.

We can evaluate each person as an individual, and make decisions accordingly. That's the smart move anyway. There's no reason to be negative. And no true advantage.

I remember sitting in a pew in a Baptist Church in North Dakota, singing "Jesus loves the little children. All the children of the world. Red and yellow. Black and white. They are precious in His sight."

In the late Sixties I renewed my passion for sewing, a demonstration of the uncharted power of genetics. I am my mother's daughter!

Many a night, after the children were asleep in bed, I sewed until dawn, because it was so relaxing for me. Not too smart, I guess, although I must have needed the creative outlet. The next day, I'd be exhausted, because I had no sleep, and five active children to nurture.

One night my husband was out at Pine Hills Country Club playing poker. It was late and I was sewing an outfit for one of the children. The TV was playing in the background.

Suddenly the news came through that Bobby Kennedy had been shot. I couldn't believe it had happened again. I called my husband and told him. Talk about reliving a nightmare!

How can we avoid this? There are so many confused and hostile people in the world. Part of the problem is that they didn't have the right advantages when they were growing up. Their situation was bad. Maybe they didn't have good parents, or maybe their own parents were beaten, or didn't have any love. Maybe a bad teacher negatively influenced them. Treat people unfairly, and that affects them the rest of their life.

Oh, I know that there are "political" reasons, and "greed" reasons for assassinations. Some people will do anything to get what they want. So much the worse for them!

The root of their evil is not knowing what's really important and what's really valuable. Anyway, the political people almost always find someone else to do the dirty work. To be willing to kill…every good person and every good religion knows that's wrong.

We in America are blessed. Affluence has given us the luxury of moving beyond primitive survival "law of the jungle" psychology. We can thoroughly analyze our relations with others.

We can see how a small act of kindness—or malice—ripples through a relationship, a family, a community, a world. Love, compassion, kindness—gifts we can give, gifts we need.

I enjoyed the Bi-Centennial celebration, because I've always felt a palpable pride in being American. I'm grateful my ancestors came here.

My grandparents were born in Germany and migrated to south Russia to avoid a war. Catherine the Great had a policy of giving land to immigrant farmers. That worked for a while, but eventually the Russian government began to levy unfair and discriminatory taxes on the wheat harvest. That's when my family left and found their way to the Dakotas, first South, and then North.

Kelly and I were thrilled by the tall ships, fireworks, and memorial services that marked America's two hundredth birthday. Even the most cynical and jaded persons—which we definitely are not—could not help but be reminded that America has always been a land of free choice and fair play.

Intolerance and bigotry—to put it quite simply—have no place in the America I love.

I guess that's a good reason to respect small town life. People are known, and held accountable for their words and actions. This has a tendency to upgrade behavior. It's no accident that the worst people feel compelled to wear sheets over their head.

Another element of small town life is neighbor helping neighbor. Volunteering for community service is routine.

My life has been no different. Years ago, I volunteered to head up the Marseilles Red Cross, and also was active in the church, including organizing a junior choir.

My musical background was sparse, true, but I had a strong feeling for the benefits of preparation and performance.

The choir members were all teenagers, including our children. Being of that age and ilk, their interest in practicing was intermittent.

To keep them active and interested, I organized sledding parties, house parties, and the like. Hot chocolate is always a big favorite after a few hours on a cold sled.

For the house parties, I'd set up a few card tables, each with its own game. Checkers, cards, Monopoly, whatever.

One year we gave a Christmas church program, and arranged it so that even the shyest youngsters sang a solo. I had them all participate, because I knew that once they conquered their fears and performed publicly, the benefits would last them forever. Literally.

Once I took our singers to see the Sound of Music performed in La Salle. Unfortunately, I forgot to switch off the car lights. The battery went dead. And there I was in a station wagon piled full of kids.

I didn't know what I was going to do, but I wasn't worried. Not in the least. I guarantee you, though, that I invoked prayer to protect those kids. Someone with jumper cables "happened" by, and stopped, powered us up, and sent us on our way.

Now if you don't see that as a demonstration of the power of prayer, maybe you need to reconsider how you're living your life.

Even before help arrived, while we were trying unsuccessfully to coax sufficient power from the battery to start the car, I was not concerned about the children's parents being upset with me. I knew them all well, and we trusted each other.

The members of my church bestowed a great honor upon me in 1983. They elected me their first female moderator. In our church, the moderator is in charge.

You never know whether you deserve something like that or not. All you can do is appreciate the trust, remind yourself of the many others who could handle the job better, and then simply concentrate on everything that needs to be done.

The main responsibility of a moderator is to serve on all the church committees, from the main ones (like the trustees), to the smaller ones, still important to the congregation (like the altar committee).

After I accepted the job, I learned that the responsibility for giving a sermon shifted to me when the minister was unable to serve.

Since the latter didn't seem likely, I didn't give it too much thought.

Then one Sunday morning, with the minister on vacation, the scheduled substitute broke her leg. Suddenly what had seemed humorous when theoretical now loomed real and imminent.

You can bet my sermon was quite brief that day. I spoke on the idea of positive thinking, and it went something like this:

"When you get up in the morning, you have a choice. You can step out of bed and choose to be miserable, and make other people miserable. Or you can decide to be happy and make other people happy. No one makes this choice but you. It's important to make the right decision. It's unhealthy to think bad thoughts about others, and it's healthy to think good ones."

Speaking of church stories, here is my favorite.

In our early days in Marseilles, as I have indicated, the town had many small grocery stores and pharmacies. All of them allowed their customers to charge their purchases, and settle their accounts on a monthly basis. We all knew each other, so this was not a risky business practice.

When our children were young, it was normal for us to give one or more a grocery list, and send them to the nearest store, a couple blocks from the house. The grocer would fill the order, and then the children always said (as they had been instructed), "Charge it to Dr. Sutton."

One Sunday morning our family was attending church, where the children always conducted themselves reasonably well. We had a rule that if you didn't behave in church, you had to spend an hour in your room when you got home. They dreaded that punishment.

Anyway, our five children were sitting in a row. Along came Bud Spencer with the collection plate. When it passed by Ruth (she was five at the time), she said, in a loud voice, "Charge it to Dr. Sutton."

The congregation roared. Funny, yes, yet in her own unique way Ruth had spontaneously created a moment of joyous fellowship for our church.

Now days, I only serve on one committee—Altar. It's not a big job. We organize two Sunday dinners a year. I can't say I really work hard, but I do try to help with donations. My company is able to provide food, like when we have our chicken-on-biscuit Sunday brunch.

One wonderful aspect of church life is that we all do what we can…and everyone's quality of life improves. A rising tide lifts all boats.

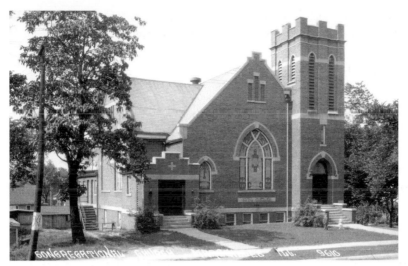

The First Congregational Church of Marseilles

As my children grew, they—and their choir friends—became less and less interested in singing together. The children's choir is now officially extinct.

Worse, it seems church has a diminishing appeal for teenagers. That can't be good, even though I realize that more and more people are finding their own private paths to God. I don't know how many are teenagers, though.

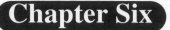

Chapter Six

D r. Sutton—okay, Kelly (really Herman Kelly)—routinely made house calls before going to his office to see his other patients. In those days, people just plain expected a doctor to come to them.

Often the at-home person in need of treatment was elderly, and living with their family. In those days, the idea of going to an Emergency Room when you were sick or injured was only marginally relevant in Marseilles and Ottawa.

We didn't have an ambulance. The local undertaker could transport someone who needed to go to the hospital, but that was a ride nobody liked.

Ottawa Hospital had an emergency room, and if one of his patients showed up there, Kelly was called in to handle the treatment.

It was not unusual for him to spend all night at the hospital with his patients, and then come home and take a short nap before going to the office and putting in a full day. He told me that once he got busy, he didn't think about the lack of sleep. "I never even felt tired," he reported. "There wasn't time. My patients depended on me."

Kelly has a lot of energy. One more reason we are a match.

No doubt my husband practiced medicine in an extraordinary time. In those days, the doctor and the patient had a more personal relationship. He had an opportunity to develop a sense of the total person. Don't think that doesn't help!

One afternoon our clinic received a call from a woman working at a dance bar type of place in a nearby town. Okay, a strip joint, and she was a stripper.

The poor girl had a huge abscessed boil on her butt, and it was hindering her work. In fact, she felt her job was in danger, and she needed the money. What could she do?

We had her come into the clinic and Kelly opened the abscess right there in our office. He bandaged the affected area, and suggested to the woman that she go to the dime store and purchase some kind of stick-on decorative item. Which she did. Probably gave her act a bit of novelty.

Of course, we didn't go to see her perform—well, I didn't, for sure. Maybe Kelly did. I don't think so.

I remember when Kelly had a young high school student come to his clinic for the first time. The boy was in high school and suffering from serious hearing loss.

During his examination, Kelly and his physician's assistant, Rod Full, found two round lumps of tin foil in each ear. Apparently, when the young fellow was in fourth grade, he developed the habit of storing foil in his ears.

What did he say when Kelly removed the remnants?

"I can hear now."

Another time Kelly soothed (by phone) one of his patients whose infant son (in diapers) had swallowed a penny.

"Don't worry," advised Kelly. "It will come through eventually. If it doesn't, we'll have to do something, but I think he will pass it. Keep checking his stool and let me know."

A few days later the father called to excitedly proclaim, "It came through, but it was a dime! What should I do now?"

Kelly's reply: "Give him another penny."

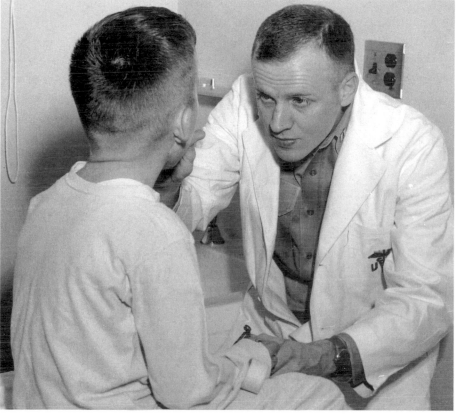

Young Dr. Sutton

My husband's natural wit helped him relax his patients. A funny remark can reduce tension, cut through the fog of fear and pain, and remind a patient that he trusts his doctor.

Once a woman came into the clinic with a blemish on her arm.

Kelly saw at a glance it was cancerous. She asked if he was going to take a sample for a biopsy. He told her he was going to remove the effected area—plus a safety perimeter—and send it to the lab for testing.

So he did. The entire procedure, including diagnosis and preparation, took less than a half-hour. Sure enough, the report came back affirming the diagnosis, and the cure.

By the time Kelly informed her of her danger, it was over.

Oh, by the way, the entire cost: $39.

Every Christmas, we went through our past due accounts. If people owed us money, we tried to think why. Maybe we knew a good reason. For example, perhaps the husband had lost his job, or a family had many children to feed.

We selected one or two of the families each year, and called them to say "Merry Christmas," and tell them they no longer owed us money. Their appreciation for our gesture filled us with far more happiness than money can ever buy.

In the latter part of his practice, we sent a card of congratulations and a small check to every patient graduating from high school. The "thank you" letters and comments we received told us how much this unexpected support was appreciated.

Kelly also enjoyed learning about who in town was related to whom. Sometimes a whole family would come in with one of their own who needed treatment. He thought it helpful to gain an understanding of their genealogy, and thus would probe (in a gentle way) their family tree. He felt this general knowledge gave him a perspective which enabled superior treatment.

Medicine did not have much information about gene transmission at that point in time, although the work of Gregor Mendel was well known. Research was being done in the 50s, 60s, and 70s, and discoveries were made, but this was a time of speculation rather than knowledge.

Mendel, an Augustinian Monk who lived in the 19th century, did "generation to generation" research with peas and with mice. His work became the foundation for modern genetics. He came to some conclusions about hereditary patterns that are quite useful for the modern parent.

For example, did you know each parent transmits only half of her or his hereditary factors to each offspring? And each child inherits a different "bundle?"

That explains a lot about sibling variance, as far as I'm concerned.

I'm very proud of the way Kelly's mind works. He doesn't do things by rote or routine. My husband is a thinker. He evaluates facts and possibilities. It's easy to look back, and say, "Don't let the patient lose blood." But a doctor trying to apply practical medicine in the 15th century normally would have been guided by "conventional wisdom" that advocated bloodletting.

I'm sure that if Dr. Sutton had been practicing then, he would have thought something like this: "Hmm. If someone is wounded, maybe we should try to stop the bleeding. It seems like a person gets weaker when losing blood. I don't see the wisdom of blood-letting." And he wouldn't have gone along with the trend. No barber pole for him!

Kelly is a conservative doctor—witness his approach to the use of estrogen by female menopausal patients. He thought menopause was a natural process. To interfere with its normal course was risky. Thus, disagreeing with the theory of the treatment, he never put a patient on estrogen.

The drug salespeople place heavy pressure on doctors, wanting them to prescribe certain products. This is a problem for medicine because it is an attempt to substitute the profit motive for dispassionate judgment.

Kelly would never allow sales logic to determine his treatment approach. He always analyzed the situation, both in making the diagnosis, and in carrying out the treatment. His medical approach was pure and true. "How can I help?"

When he grabbed the chart and walked through the door to see the next patient, he was focused and attentive to the situation at hand. It didn't matter whether the patient was on public aid, or had an outstanding bill. I know for sure his only objective was healing. No question about it.

Incidentally, new studies have come out recently, and they confirm his thinking about estrogen. Many women who used it to ease the pains of menopause must now worry about a significantly increased susceptibility to cancer.

(The justifiably happy wife says) my husband was about 50 years ahead of his time on that one. I wish every woman had been his patient.

I'm proud to be a Sutton.

Kelly once treated 113 patients in a single day, including hospital and house calls. This in a town with a population of 5,000. He estimates he has delivered more than two thousand babies into this wonderful world.

In a way, Dr. Sutton is a modern version of the Dodge City doctor depicted in the television series "Gunsmoke." One of the treats of watching that program is seeing Doc Adams practice medicine in what many might consider a primitive era. From our modern perspective, it is easier today to make a diagnosis and affect a healing.

Yet Doc Adams did very well by his patients because he exercised his thinking rights. He observed, he examined, he thought, and he doctored. I believe that's how someone from the 22nd century would evaluate Kelly's work.

Naturally, I'm not this effusive to his face. In fact, I always tell people, especially if he's around, that I married my husband because the name "Seattle Sutton" sounded good. My teasing doesn't have much effect, because after nearly 50 years of marriage, five children, and 14 grandchildren, I don't think he cares "why" I married him.

Kelly's dry sense of humor manifests itself in certain comments—some of them could be taken as a little rude—that he gets by with because they make people laugh. Humor can heal depression, you know. If you get the joke.

I love to laugh, but I'm a little more serious than Kelly. Many times, I fall in the category of people who don't understand his sense of humor.

When his relatives visit, or his high school classmates, such as Ted Myrna and Floyd Kingston, I enjoy sitting in the background and hearing them talk about their high school experiences in Eldorado. They reminiscence and laugh, tell jokes and laugh, look at each other funny and laugh. I'm not very good at telling jokes, but I like to hear them.

One evening, in 1969, a group of us were sitting around having a good time, laughing (of course), and playing cards. Happy companions.

One of our friends told a joke. He finished with the punch line: "That's life." He said it…and died.

My husband and I tried to save him. Kelly ran to the car and got his medical bag. We gave him CPR. We could not revive him.

As we shared our grief for our friend, a general consensus formed—the deceased had worked too hard. I couldn't help thinking about my husband, "My goodness, he also is overworked."

Kelly had a lot of confidence in his ability to help his patients heal. He enjoyed his work, and showed no sign of weakness, but my concern about the general toll his long hours might be taking on his health was real.

The clincher (for me) came a few days later when my husband, scheduled to be a pallbearer for our departed friend, got tied up with an emergency at the hospital, and missed the funeral.

I decided I would do everything I could to help reduce his workload. He ran his practice the old-fashioned way—doing everything himself—and didn't even have a nurse in his office at that time.

Our youngest child, Sarah, was in third grade, so I knew I could organize our home while they were all in school. I told Kelly, "Look, I've been thinking about helping you in the office." He offered no resistance, having come to the same conclusion.

"Yes, maybe for an hour or two a day." Well, that "hour or two" quickly turned into something more than full time, as we knew it would. My normal day soon consisted of getting the kids ready and off to school, doing a few chores around the house and yard, and arriving in the office by 10 a.m.

Kelly didn't like any part of running the business aspect of his medical practice, and I realized if I took that load he could concentrate on taking care of his patients—which he loved.

In order to help him, I had to sort out my priorities, which is why I gave up sewing and some of my volunteer work.

I began to run the business, learning on the job, reading everything I could find. Medical Economics magazine was especially helpful. Eventually I learned enough to incorporate the business, establish a profit sharing plan, and much more.

More than once, as I sat at the desk, I remembered that my mother did the bookkeeping while my dad did the selling. The apple doesn't fall far from the tree.

Once I asked Kelly how many people he had seen that day who would not require his medical attention if they had always eaten a proper, healthy, well-balanced diet.

His answer: "Of the approximately 40 people who came in today, probably ninety per cent."

Ninety per cent! That shows the importance of healthy eating.

People can get by with junk food for a while, especially teenagers. After a certain amount of time, though, the effects become visible.

The same is true for eating food containing dyes. Large amounts of food dyes, especially "Red 40," can cause bladder cancer in mice. Yellow 5 & 6, and Blue 1 & 2 may also be detrimental to the human body. This is verified by scientific experiment. Well, if it causes cancer in mice, are people also at risk? Likely.

Read the label! Please. And teach your children to do the same. Avoid things like artificial sweeteners, questionable additives, and food dyes. Every one of these could be bad for young and old alike. Their negative effects damage people. You, dear reader, are no exception.

We seldom gave our children vitamins, despite the fact that Kelly received a constant stream of samples in cute containers. Sometimes the children were attracted to the vitamins because of the bottles, and we'd let them try, but that was always limited and temporary.

The children knew their way around the new clinic. We taught them to file charts, and draw blood. I think this gave the girls confidence they could be nurses.

Kelly liked to show Paula a picture of the effects of an ailment, and then bring her into the examination room to see them on a real-life patient. No doubt he was preparing her for a medical career.

Anyone can get sick, despite a lifetime of healthy eating and taking good care of themselves. That's an unfortunate aspect of life. My husband had only missed one day of work in 40 years He was never, ever, sick.

After a happy vacation in Mexico with four other couples, we came home feeling good. Two days later Kelly collapsed while in the bathroom.

Oh, it pains me to remember. He could barely move enough to open the door and call me. I caught him as he was leaning over the sink, about to fall.

I called the ambulance. It arrived quickly, though the interval seemed forever. We raced to the hospital. Kelly was bleeding rectally. Following bowel surgery, he developed peritonitis, with a number of complications.

Five days after this first operation, his doctors decided he had to have a colostomy. I knew he might not survive. So did my daughters. They are nurses, after all. Chris and Pete also fully understood the situation.

Paula, who always put her whole heart into every situation, and accepts every challenge, is the most empathic and sensitive of our children. She tearfully told me she had "never taken care of any patient as sick as dad who lived."

Her statement held an ominous meaning, because hospital management where she worked, noting her exceptional sensitivity and dedication, routinely assigns her to nurse seriously ill patients.

For days, her tears fell like winter rain. Every morning we checked her purse to make sure she had a new supply of Kleenex. Believe it or not, that little tease helped.

Kelly's medical situation reached such a dire strait that our daughter Sarah asked a friend of the family, Father Jim Curtin, to anoint him with the Sacrament for the Sick, and administer the last rites. Oh dear!

My beloved husband almost didn't make it through his second surgery. The doctors performed the colostomy and left the skin of his abdomen open to aid in his healing.

Kelly was in Intensive Care for 17 days. He doesn't remember that his sons visited from Washington and California.

The Marseilles priest, Fr. Bo Schmitt, dropped by to tell us that many of his parishioners were praying for Kelly. My husband and I are members of the First Congregational Church of Marseilles, and we were especially grateful for Catholic support. We told the priest we needed all the prayers we could get, and it didn't matter which religion.

Our minister, Rev. Ron Seider, visited our family at the hospital almost every day, and was very supportive with his encouragement and prayers.

After the second surgery, the boys headed back home, leaving their three nurse sisters to tend Kelly around the clock. The surgeon, Dr. Joseph Kokoszka, called the girls, "the Suttonettes."

During the times my husband had worked at the hospital in Ottawa, his calm demeanor earned him friends and respect. Whether he was in surgery, or passing someone in the hall, he never failed to be polite and considerate.

In his illness, janitors came to wish him well, and so did physicians, and staff, and former patients. They respected Kelly, and cared about him.

My thought every day was "it's nothing malignant, and it'll be all right if we can get him through this."

That's what we did. One day at a time.

Finally, he was moved from intensive care to the floor. A few days later, we took him home, though he couldn't walk or stand erect. I placed a hospital bed in our family room, and cancelled all my other engagements.

When the home nurse told him, "We're going to teach you how to change your dressing (on the open wound) and your colostomy bag,"

Kelly responded, "No, you're not." He pointed at me. "She'll do it."

So I was in charge of that. I didn't mind.

Twice in nine months circumstances forced him to manage the bag change himself. Afterwards, he gave his report, "I made a big mess." As if I didn't know.

It wasn't easy. Yet he's psychologically strong. He didn't get discouraged. That helped immensely.

When Kelly learned how devoted his daughters had been during his illness, he nodded his head and remarked, "You owed me. I paid for your education."

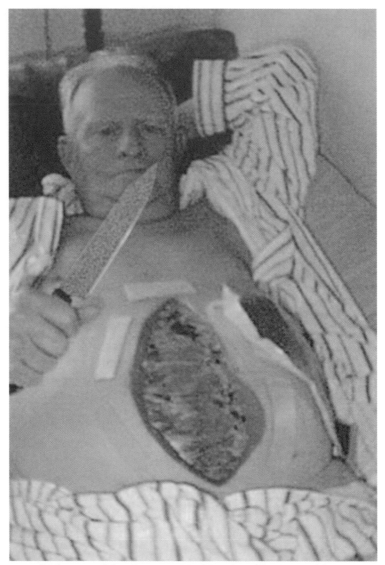

Kelly sent this photo to his friends with the caption,
"You should see the other guy"

During the night, I slept on a nearby sofa so I could hear if he needed me. Very early one morning he tried to sit in the chair beside his bed without my help. He didn't make it, and sank to the floor. That's when he called for me.

We struggled to get him at least to a kneeling position, but I was not strong enough. I couldn't do it! We both started laughing because the situation seemed…well, funny.

I looked at the clock and realized that our friend Dick Naretty almost always got out of bed by 4 a.m. to exercise and lift weights. I phoned Dick for help.

He made it to our house within five minutes, and lifted my husband onto the bed like it was nothing.

What a relief! Thank God for friends. Amen!

When Kelly and I told the story to friends, we laughed again. Our shared laughter relieved me, because I could see that my husband was not becoming discouraged.

He received many get-well cards from friends, patients, and many, many people from Marseilles and Ottawa. I couldn't fit them all on the big sideboard in the living room.

Eight months later, he had gained enough strength to enable us to go on trips. We even drove all the way down to Texas to surprise our grandson Reece on his 16th birthday.

We had to find large bathrooms—like in 7-11s or places like that, so I could go with him and help. That worked out fine.

He kept getting better and better. His weight had dropped to 129 pounds from his normal 165, and he started to gain again, finally stabilizing at 155.

Nine months after his collapse in our bathroom, the doctors sent Kelly to the University of Illinois Medical Center (where he had received his medical education). His colostomy was reversed, and the doctors inserted mesh to close his abdomen. He's been doing well ever since.

I don't think there were many minutes in a day that I didn't have the thought that I couldn't go on if I lost him. I am so glad he's still around. We're very fortunate that he survived. Through sickness and health, that's right, we've been two people whom God has joined together.

To make sure a marriage is not "put asunder" requires that both parties expect a lot from each other, and also give a lot.

What does this mean as a practical matter? First and foremost, forgive and forget the "little" things. If you become angry and upset, have the patience to allow time to work its magic.

Most importantly, a wife and husband must communicate. If one partner is unhappy, it's important that the other knows why, and cares.

In most families, women are the best communicators. I always took it as my responsibility to make sure the important issues were well-discussed. Kelly might not have shared my feelings about the value of communication, and placed the burden on my shoulders, but that's okay.

Now I see that he's very proud of how well our children, and their spouses, and our grandchildren communicate, and get along, and want to be with each other. Speaking from the perspective of our family's matriarch and patriarch, that's one of our most satisfying accomplishments.

After Dr. Sutton quit his practice, every morning he would wake up and announce, "Today I fixed so-and-so's fractured leg." He would dream about his patients just about every night.

When he became ill, his mind must have been busy elsewhere, because he ceased to have such dreams. As soon as he recovered, they started again.

Kelly and I have never argued about money. He always trusted my judgment on spending...and I trusted his. We are both finacially cautious.

Now he'll notice something when we're out shopping, and say, "My gosh, that is so expensive." My answer is always, "Kelly, if you can't keep up with inflation, that's a sure sign you're getting old."

Inflation is a fact of commerce. As we get older, things cost more, even if they are not as nice. We remember, "Back when I was a child, this is what it cost." It's okay to talk about that once in a while, but if you make a big issue of it, you're really getting old.

Another sign of age, as we all know, is forgetting things. Did I already tell you this?

Then there are the times of being "not very smart." Sure, as we get older, we do dumb things. We might forget our keys, for example. But age can also bring wisdom, and we can devise a plan that makes it easier to find them. We can always leave them in the same place, for example. There's no reason to be frustrated by aging.

Frustration is also the real enemy of a happy marriage. The danger is that you might take your frustration out on your spouse. We have a rule against that in the Sutton household.

Our 50th wedding anniversary is almost here. Wow!

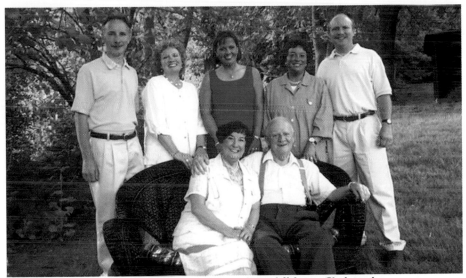
My husband and I with our five children, Christopher,
Paula, Sarah, Ruth, and Peter

"Kelly," I mused, "Can you believe we'll be married fifty years?"
His ultra-romantic answer? "Yes, and I still have all my teeth!"

So funny. He never fails to speak what's on his mind. And that
afternoon he had dental work done. He hates going to the dentist.

Sure, I expected he might make a romantic comment, but when
you live with someone for almost fifty years, you understand what is
hard, and what is easy. And what they don't like doing.

"Did the dentist hurt you?"

"No, but they make you lie down, and open your mouth, and then
they attack you and don't let up until the job is done."

Well, I repeatedly have told my husband that, if I could go to the
dentist for him, I would. Some things, no matter how strong the love,
can't be helped.

I don't know if my husband will give me a gift for our fiftieth.
It's certainly not necessary (just like an engagement ring). However,
I very much appreciated the ring he gave me for our twenty-fifth
anniversary.

When you've been married a long time, there's really nothing new
to give or get. But I truly appreciate that sometimes when he goes
out to purchase some staples at the grocery store, he buys a bunch of
really nice red radishes, and cleans them for me. He tells me "that's
instead of red roses."

He knows how much I love good red radishes. Living proof you
can give "gifts of love" without spending a lot of money. If he
bought me clothing, chances are it would hang in the closet.

Red radishes are perfect.

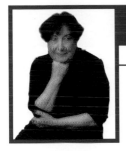

Use Your Thinking Rights!

FAD & GIMMICK DIETS

Most people are totally frustrated when they try to begin a calorie-controlled diet to lose weight. To do it right takes planning, shopping, cooking, calorie calculating; and all this requires time.

These diet elements are not willpower friendly. Frustration often leads to postponement, or quitting.

It's easy to be tempted by a fad diet, given these conditions. But this usually makes the situation worse.

Short-term weight loss is the lure of a typical gimmick diet. Permanent weight loss is the quality of a healthy diet—which should last and extend—one's lifetime.

A fad diet asks you to eat in a way no one can sustain. Weight losses are promised, and perhaps momentarily achieved, but, ultimately, the consumer is misled. Any change in eating habits is not permanent. Neither are the results.

For example, during the relatively short time a person could be allowed to use it, the liquid diet resulted in a loss of weight. No choices were involved and calorie intake was strictly controlled.

These two characteristics are the basics of any workable weight loss formula. We use them both at Seattle Sutton's Healthy Eating, except we apply them via a balanced and healthy menu, and a wide variety of meals. That's the bedrock of our longevity and our success—and how we help people.

Fad diets, on the other hand, have no chance of working. They may provide temporary weight loss, but this is an illusion. The dieter will almost always gain every pound back (and quite likely more) once the previous eating pattern is resumed.

The most important aspect of a diet is its lifespan, which should coincide with that of the dieter. When you consider going on a diet, you should use your thinking rights, and ask yourself, "Can I eat this way the rest of my life?"

If the answer is yes, there's no need to guess, the diet is right.

If the answer is no, that way don't go, the diet is wrong.

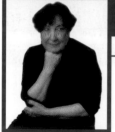

In general, Americans eat too much fat. Big surprise.

A healthy intake of fat should be 30% or less of a person's daily calories. Fewer than ten percent of total fat calories should come from saturated fats. Yet most Americans consume more than this recommendation.

A high fat diet can lead to colon cancer and obesity, with all its attendant dangers. But as many doctors and dieticians warn the public to lower its fat intake, a sort of knee jerk reaction is taking place. Some people reason that if low fat is good, no fat must be better. Talk about an urban myth!

Make no mistake. The body needs fat for hair, skin, and nutriment.

The trick is to reduce fat without eliminating it. It may help to remember that fats are heavy with calories. Nine per gram.

Reducing the intake of fat can be a way to automatically reduce calories as long as dieters are careful not to consume more calories elsewhere.

One can't eat a whole box of non-fat cookies, for example, and still lose weight. Make no mistake. Non-fat cookies contain calories.

Science divides fat into two groups, "good" and "bad." Both "kinds" have the dreaded nine calories per gram.

"Good" is found in vegetable oils, including olive oil. Good is unsaturated, whether poly or mono. "Bad" is animal fat, and anything hydrogenated, such as saturated and trans fat, both of which stick to arteries.

The term "hydrogenated" describes the process of "blowing" hydrogen gas into vegetable oil. The latter, by itself, is "good." But hydrogenation solidifies it and creates trans fat. One example is margarine. A smart goal: choose a margarine low in trans fats.

Cutting down on bad fat is common sense. Use your thinking rights!

By the way, Seattle Sutton's Healthy Eating meal plans contain about 22% of total calories from fat, and less than 7% of total calories from saturated fats.

Did a physician advise you to go on a low carb diet? High protein or high fat? I'd switch doctors. The low carb diet is simply another fad. I don't feel it is a healthy, well-balanced way of eating.

Don't misunderstand me. I know that high protein diets can lead to weight loss because protein calories are energy-expensive for the body to burn. Protein is hard to break down, and therefore the body uses more calories during digestion and metabolism.

High protein diets generally result in weight loss over a six-month period, but after a year, results tend to dissipate, and soon there is no difference between a moderate carbohydrate diet and a low carbohydrate diet.

Even without going on a low carb diet, Americans in general eat twice as much protein as necessary. Any further increase could add stress to our kidneys and livers. This is especially a problem for the elderly and the diabetic.

To date, no major health care organization embraces the high protein diets, and most denounce them. A recent study done by Duke University, seemingly promoting the Atkins Diet, is clouded because it turned out to be sponsored by the Atkins Foundation.

Here's an insightful quote from a Chicago Tribune editorial:

"We're from the old school that's suspicious of the latest diet crazes in general, preferring a more common-sense approach. Give up an abundance of fruits and vegetables? Sorry, but you'll have to peel our cold, dead hands from that Granny Smith apple.

"As Linda Van Horn, professor of preventive medicine at Northwestern's Feinberg School of Medicine, says: 'There's never been a study ever conducted that says fruits and vegetables are bad for you. Quite the contrary.'"

(Continued)

Another study, released in January of 2004, claimed people could lose weight by eating a high carbohydrate and low fat diet, just the opposite of the low carb method. I suppose it's not surprising that something as radical as a low carb diet would spur a compensatory rival.

I strongly recommend the common sense, scientific approach: a healthy, balanced diet in line with one hundred years of fair-minded mainstream nutrition research. Need I repeat calories in vs. calories out?

A successful diet cannot be measured by initial weight loss alone. The criteria must be permanent fat loss achieved in a healthy way. Who among us honestly feels a low carb plan is something to stick with for the rest of our life?

A restrictive diet, eliminating certain foods or food groups, demonstrates the worst failure rate over time. A low carb diet essentially discards several foods and food groups.

Is this healthy? Reason says no.

The Atkins people have not published a single study showing the long-term effects of his diet on heart health. Considering the diet has been around since the 70s, they certainly have had ample time to do so.

It appears that many companies attempt to confuse the public. Use your thinking rights.

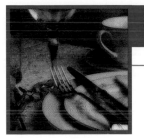

(MONDAY:)
Dinner: LEMON PEPPER LOAF

A tasty combination of a lemon pepper loaf, twice baked potato and cooked spinach, served with steamed apples with cinnamon and nutmeg all to remind you of grandma's cooking.

(TUESDAY:)
Breakfast: DELICIOUS RAISIN BISCUIT

With fresh fruit.

Lunch: QUICHE & SPINACH SALAD

A light mushroom crust filled with a blend of "no-cholesterol" eggs, cheeses and diced scallions, accompanied by fresh spinach leaves with zesty dressing.

Dinner: GARDEN PATTY

Veggie patty on a poppy seed bun, served with old fashioned, hearty potato soup, tomato juice, and lemon cookies.

(WEDNESDAY:)
Breakfast: HOMESTYLE FRENCH TOAST

Covered with spiced apple topping. Served with veggie links.

Lunch: SALSA CHICKEN SANDWICH

A seasoned broiled chicken breast topped with salsa on a fresh baked roll, served with seasonal fruit.

Dinner: ORANGE ROUGHY

A baked fillet of orange roughy topped with tomato, onion and celery bits and sprinkled with paprika, served on a bed of long grain wild rice and accompanied by parsleyed carrots.

(THURSDAY:)
Breakfast: ORANGE APPLE STRUDEL

With tangy orange sauce and grapefruit juice.

Lunch: POCKET PITA

A slice of aged Swiss cheese, garbanzo beans and fresh garden greens all tucked in a whole wheat pita pocket with a refreshing yogurt cucumber dressing and petite orange.

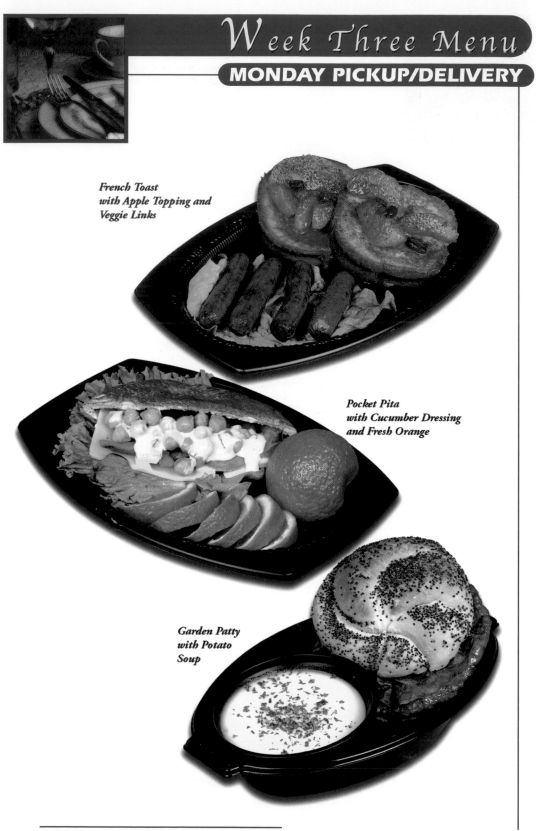

*French Toast
with Apple Topping and
Veggie Links*

*Pocket Pita
with Cucumber Dressing
and Fresh Orange*

*Garden Patty
with Potato
Soup*

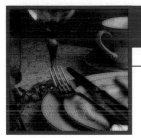

(THURSDAY:)

Dinner: SWEET & SOUR ORIENTAL ENTREE

Fried rice topped with pieces of meat, pineapple, vegetables and water chestnuts in a sweet and sour demi glaze. This meal includes a vegetable egg roll and fortune cookie.

(FRIDAY:)

Breakfast: BREAKFAST WRAP WITH SALSA

Lunch: EUROPEAN LUNCH

Low fat cottage cheese with a healthy variety of fruits, served with cinnamon flatbread.

Dinner: HEIRLOOM RAVIOLI

Cheese stuffed ravioli smothered with a hearty tomato sauce with
healthful broccoli spears and garlic toast.

(SATURDAY:)

Breakfast: CLASSIC CINNAMON APPLE OATMEAL

With an english muffin, and fruit spread.

Lunch: BOUNTIFUL BARLEY SOUP

Variations of vegetables, barley and meat kettle-simmered to a pleasing
flavor with oyster crackers and a small apple.

Dinner: BOCA BURGER

The popular meatless burger with garnish, on a whole wheat hamburger bun, served with our special homestyle baked beans and delicious rice pudding.

(SUNDAY:)

Breakfast: FRUIT AND SSHE'S VERY OWN GRANOLA

Lunch: TORTELLINI VEGETABLE SOUP

A hearty soup of tortellini and garden fresh vegetables simmered in a rich broth, accompanied by a fresh spinach salad with flavorful dressing and a rye bun.

Dinner: SPAGHETTI WITH MEAT SAUCE

A Seattle Sutton specialty. Chunky meat sauce on top of pasta, accompanied by our best celery cheese bake and spiced peach.

(MONDAY:)

Breakfast: DELICATE CARROT MUFFIN

And iron rich plump yellow raisins.

Lunch: RADIATTORE PASTA SALAD

A unique luncheon of pasta with terrific taste due to a blend of tasty ingredients, served with a miniature peanut snack and refreshing apricot nectar.

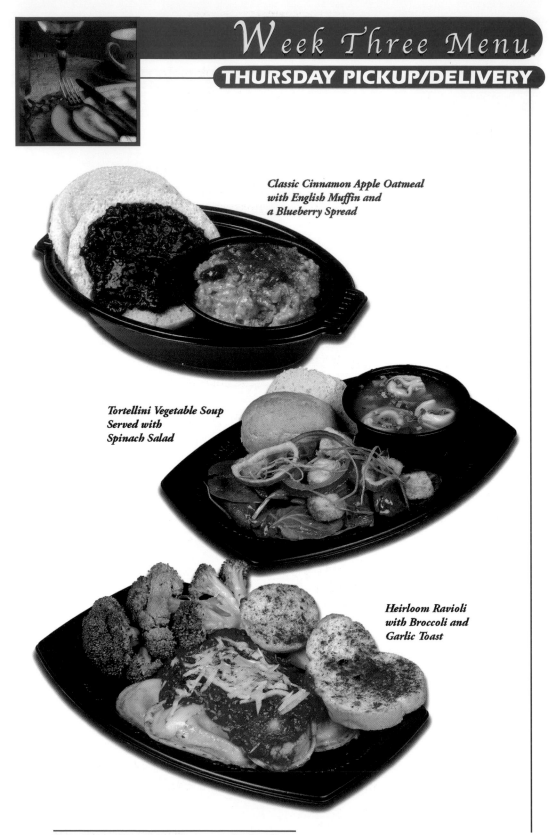

Classic Cinnamon Apple Oatmeal with English Muffin and a Blueberry Spread

Tortellini Vegetable Soup Served with Spinach Salad

Heirloom Ravioli with Broccoli and Garlic Toast

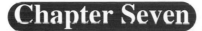

Chapter Seven

Thank you for allowing me to shuck the limits of chronology when I think it appropriate. As the book progresses, I'll be doing it more and more. Including right now.

Being a parent is such an essential part of my self-definition. I want to reach into my purse and show you a few pictures of my children and grandchildren.

What proud mother—and grandmother—wouldn't?

Parenthood is the greatest responsibility, and the greatest challenge. It is a never-ending final examination, requiring the constant practical application of everything a parent knows, hopes, fears, believes, and is.

Here's an apt quote from Dorothy Corkille Briggs: "The psychological climate that produces the freely creative productive child is made up of precisely the same ingredients that compose the climate of love."

Children will turn out to be successful, well-balanced adults if they are raised with lots of love. Love's absence, on the other hand, saddles a child with difficult burdens that delay—and sometimes derail—progress toward happiness.

Fortunately, most basic parenting advice I have ever received—by word or example—is to give my children lots of love, and make sure they know they are really, truly, unquestionably loved.

When the fact of love is established beyond doubt in a child's mind, the parents can do what is necessary—even use strict discipline. If the same child does not know his parents care about him, being criticized and corrected can easily erode self-confidence.

If you haven't laid a foundation of love for your children, if they have any question about your feelings, discipline can seem like rejection. But if you really care about them, and they know it for certain, then you can be as strict as necessary, with confidence you are doing the right thing.

While the children were growing up, I always made them aware when I didn't approve of what they were doing. That's important. I know I yelled at them when I became frustrated. I felt I could really go at that with strong fervor, because I also knew that they knew they were loved.

Strict discipline may meet a particular need. But it is so much better to reward for good behavior than to punish for bad. When our children were exceptionally good (those hallowed times!), they were praised and rewarded.

One credo I made sure to follow: Don't just tell them what to do (clean their room, for instance), show them! Kelly and I always made sure they knew our expectations, especially about how to treat and respect each other.

Fortunate is the family that raises its children in a small town. "It takes a village" is not just a political catch phrase. The primary advantage is that everyone cares—and knows—about everyone else.

Some people think of this as negative. I understand, but feel compelled to point out a redeeming positive.

Almost everyone in Marseilles helped our children, including members of our church, our friends, our children's friends, their teachers…the list goes on.

A network of goodness surrounded Chris, Paula, Peter, Ruth, and Sarah. Love was their window to the world, shaping the way they perceived and evaluated their circumstances, and made their choices. This helped them become good, honest people.

One teacher, for example, can be a positive life-long influence on a child. I remember my eighth grade teacher, Miss Englehart, complimenting me on the quality of my work. She reinforced the confidence my parents had given me. It carried forward. I still remember her.

My friend Kathy Naretty is a great teacher. She never had any children of her own, yet I consider her an outstanding parent. She was thoughtful and conscientious about helping her students and influencing them to lead a loving, self-expressive life. Her former students often return to Kathy, and say, "You were an excellent teacher. I remember many things you taught us. They've helped me throughout my life."

When we encounter a child—related or not—we can treat them well, and be a good and lasting influence. I'm grateful to all who were that way with mine.

Kelly and I both believe that good parents pay quality attention to their children. This precept was challenged when I started to help out in the office. Though they were all in school, the extra work I was doing could have posed a threat.

I wasn't going to neglect the children. I decided to establish a regime that would benefit them, and maintain our closeness as a family.

We laid down the rules. They were to entertain no company until we came home. As soon as they returned from school, they were to go to the refrigerator door and check the list of chores—some for each of them. They were to do nothing else until their jobs were finished. I'm sure that many times they came home hoping the list would be non-existent, or at least short.

The children had to finish their jobs by a given deadline. We made sure they understood the consequences of non-compliance. Finish their housework—and their homework. Then have fun.

In the summer, they took turns preparing the weekday family meals. Five children—five days. Each of them was required to plan the meals for her or his day, buy the groceries (charging it to Dr. Sutton, of course), prepare the food, and clean up.

One time Peter called me at the medical office and plaintively explained his inability to complete a listed chore. "Mom, I'm making this Waldorf Salad, but there's a problem. The directions says 'fold in the mayonnaise' and the kind we have doesn't fold."

Peter's complaint became one of our family's evergreen stories, retold at many a gathering. Every family is interconnected by its unique literary fabric, tales repeated at holiday gatherings, and birthdays, and funerals, like myths passed from generation to generation sitting around stone-ringed fires, celebrating the triumphs and tragedies of tribal hunts and harvests.

I believe it is of utmost importance to hold family get-togethers and share stories as often as practical, making sure to include children and grandchildren in the circle. Not only are these occasions a positive factor for all involved, but they help create and define a sense of being an important part of a loving, valuable whole.

Our family—including grandchildren—gathers several times a year, if we can. At least once is an absolute must. It's essential for grandchildren to have roots. You can't start when they are teenagers That's too late.

You have to begin at birth. Needless to say, we used to have a houseful of high chairs and cribs. At least one grandkid was always hungry, and another was always tired.

Our grandchildren got to know each other. Now they are close friends, with mutual self-respect. We like that none of them ever complain about their cousins.

I do not think this an accident.

The reason, in my opinion, our grandchildren get along so well is that they know what Kelly and I expect. Which is: show respect for each other, just like we show respect for them, and they show respect for us.

Fault is easy to discern. Anyone can find it. With due kudos (and apologies) to Edwin Starr, I say, "Fault...what is it good for? Absolutely nothing."

It doesn't promote a good relationship. It's not a good teacher. It doesn't help anything, or anybody, including the faultfinder.

Look for the good. Forgive and forget the little things. Especially when little ones are involved.

Every child does wonderful things. Prompt a demonstration of goodness, then compliment and reward. Build a good path to increased self-esteem.

Fact: As many as 49% of all children are either born out-of-wedlock, or are unwanted. A child "feels" the meaning of the word "unwanted." Such a devastating emotion. It's not material luxuries a youngster needs. Love is the foundation of happiness.

I've never believed that gifts "spoil" children. What damages youngsters is being unfair to them, constantly criticizing them, tearing down self-esteem. It's very sad to see that. No child deserves to be treated in such a vile manner.

When our children were younger, I was involved in the school's parent-teacher association (PTA). Back then, almost every parent was.

A local woman attended one of our PTA meetings. Afterwards everyone milled around talking about this and that...general conversation. The woman in question complained in a loud voice about her son being bad, carrying on at home and in the streets, not caring about anyone else. The next day, she became quite irate when someone repeated what they had heard about her son...from the gossip chain that began with her.

That's a good lesson. If there is any little problem in the family, work it out amongst the family. Discuss it. Try to improve it. Don't criticize your own children in public. It's not going to help them. It's not going to help you.

One day Sarah walked home from junior high school, crying because her bike had been stolen. Of course, nobody in Marseilles tied up their bikes. That made the theft even worse.

At dinner that night, Sarah told us what had happened, and named the person who did it. Kelly knew the family, of course, and tried to put things in perspective for Sarah.

"That girl probably could never, ever get a bicycle, and she knew you had one for years, and so she just maybe thought, 'I'd sure like to have that,' and she took it.

"Why don't you call her and tell her you know she has the bike, and you want her to keep it."

That's what Sarah did. And she never forgot Kelly's advice. The girl's family was so large—so many children—that she was not able to afford a bike. Kelly taught Sarah—and the whole family—something valuable about sharing and forgiveness.

Sarah often remarks that it was "such a good lesson, to put yourself in another's person's shoes, to think about why someone did something to me."

Parents can so easily implant the right idea in a child. All it really takes is a good example. And it lasts a lifetime.

Paula, Ruth, Sarah, and their daughters recently joined me in Atlanta, and we all flew to the Bahamas. Ten of us—three generations—laughing constantly, happy to be together, no mother and daughter and granddaughter "issues." Simply a family bound by genuine love. It's easy. Anyone can do it. You can do it.

Our family tried to have dinner together, no matter what time Kelly came home. If he were delivering a baby, we might eat as late as 10 p.m., but we did our best to make sure we ate at the same time and table.

I think eating the evening meal together is an important aspect of family life. Kelly always kept me posted if he were to be delayed, and I'd give the children healthy snacks—fruit and vegetables mostly—while we waited.

It might seem odd eating so late. I know it did to our friends. One time a few of them came by around 9 p.m. or so, looked in the window, and saw our family at the table. They left without knocking, and told us later.

We always made sure we had intelligent discussions while we ate. It's important to talk about different topics as a family.

By the way, I seldom consulted the children about the dinner menu. I promise I always served healthy meals, and was careful to broaden their palettes. If I anticipated resistance to the introduction of a new food into their diet, I would curtail snacks during the afternoon, and announce:

"Tonight our meal is going to be served in courses."

The first food served that night would be new to them. A good example is Brussels sprouts. I didn't force them to eat, but, being hungry, they took one bite, and then another, and ended up liking the new taste more and more.

If they had been given something else to eat at the same time, they might have skipped the sprouts. In this way, they learned to

No Gimmicks 89

enjoy a variety of foods. Some of our children, to my knowledge, there's no food they don't like.

Over the years, our family established it's own unique New Year's Day dining tradition. Since this was pre-Seattle Sutton's Healthy Eating, we commenced after I finished cooking dinner.

We took our seats and filled our plates, primed for the ensuing conversation. First we reminded our children of the unbreakable rule: be honest and truthful. Then we focused our attention on one family member at a time.

Two questions were asked. The first: "How would you like so-and-so to change?" Paula might say, for example, about Chris, "Don't tease me so much."

When the others had finished giving Chris advice about how he could improve himself, a second question was posed. "What do you like best about Chris?" Everyone gave an honest answer.

We went around the table asking and answering these questions. Kelly and I were not exempt. Each of the children loved telling us how they would like us to change, and, happily, what they really liked about us as their father and mother.

While you were being critiqued, you couldn't disagree or respond. You had to listen, and wait to talk. Sometimes another child's turn would bring out something like: "She shouldn't say things like that about me because that's not true." Such a response might come in due time, but I gave total leeway to the person talking.

Kelly and I took advantage of this opportunity to tell our children how they could improve. Receptivity couldn't have been better. The children were eager to learn because they were eager to teach.

It helped them, in my opinion, understand their acts had consequences. It hammered home the truth that people remember how they are treated—the good and the bad.

By gaining an increased understanding of how others perceived them, our children couldn't help but grow. Also, it was good for them to learn to criticize responsibly and follow a negative with a positive.

I highly recommend this technique. All the important things were revealed, no matter how privately they had been previously held.

None of the children knew what comments were going to be made. I guess they worried about being criticized, recalling certain things that had been done or said, and wondering if their siblings would remember. But they were very glad to hear the good things.

Chapter Eight

Love is the essence of parenting, and respect is the essence of love. We can respect our children by helping them to learn who they are and to achieve their chosen goals. We can aid the development of their interests, and show them how their decisions shape their lives.

A parent can promote the things their children like to do, but can't just assume, "Here is something that I'm going to mold." The child has to respond.

Kelly and I could see, for example, that our two boys, Chris and Pete, were very interested in electronics. So we made them a workplace in the furnace room. We built a big counter and began to purchase Heath (component) kits for the boys.

When Chris was in eighth grade, we bought him a Heath kit containing the components of a black and white television set. My husband and I figured it would keep him busy all summer.

He assembled a functioning TV in a few weeks. Thirty-five years later, it still works!

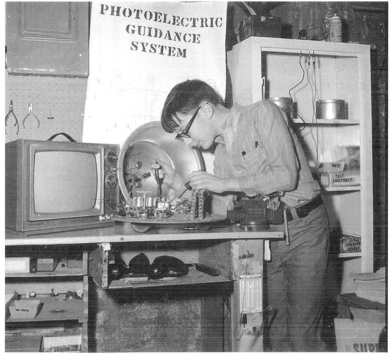

Chris in his basement workshop

I guess in a strange way that Heath kit was the equivalent of the nursing gift my mother gave me. It was clear that Chris liked electronics, so we encouraged him without commanding him.

Actually, Chris first showed his electronics flair when he was much younger, and suffering from the mumps (before vaccine). I think he was in kindergarten.

Kelly and I were on a trip to Chicago. We decided to bring Chris a present: a short-wave radio component kit. Was it a Heath? I don't remember.

We brought it home, and, soon, even with the mumps, Chris was on our roof, putting up the antenna.

We realized he had a talent, but didn't think of trying to send him away to a specialized school. We just saw to it that he had electronic things to do, when and if he wanted.

His friends frequently came over to watch him put the kits together. Eventually, he placed several chairs in a row, so they could sit and talk to him as he worked.

Chris graduated from high school in 1973, and attended the University of Illinois, where he received his master's degree in Electrical Engineering. Ever since, he's been with Hewlett-Packard/Agilent.

Peter, by the way, received his bachelor of science degree in electronics engineering technology from DeVry Institute in Chicago, took a job with a California technology company, and has worked there ever since.

Kelly and I believe it's important, no matter the size of the family, to do special things for, and with, just one child. This enhances each child's sense of individuality. Of course, we made sure every child received a turn.

As you can imagine, we had no shortage of time with all five together. It's far more difficult to arrange "solitary" outings.

When Kelly was making house calls, he sometimes took one of the children with him. Perhaps it seems like a little thing, but all five always wanted to go with their Dad.

It was a real break for me to have one of them out of the house. Having five young children disproves the old adage, "the more the merrier." At least not all the time.

Once we had to fly to Detroit, and circumstances allowed us to take only one child. Our method of selection might have been old-fashioned, but it worked.

We drew straws. Paula won, and literally vibrated with happiness. During the trip, however, she vomited frequently. I chalked it up to excitement and stress. She enjoyed the time with us and the traveling, but sometimes victory has a price. Maybe, though, it was just the airplane food.

My husband and I agree that our children's teenage years were our most fun together. Sure, they made some mistakes. One of them (neither Kelly nor I can remember which) drove our car into a telephone pole, for example. We didn't require them to be perfect.

No one expects a five-year-old to be focused. A teenager is a different challenge. A teen can be distracted, but has had more experience, and is more mature, and thus possesses more common sense.

It was a fun time for us because they were becoming little adults, and we were guiding them. I kind of cringe when I hear a parent say, "Oh, my gosh, our kids are going to be teenagers. How will we be able to stand it?" I immediately tell them what I'm writing you, that the teenage years are the best time, really the best, especially if the parents have the right mind set.

Did I ever get angry as a parent? Frustrated? Of course. Frustration is my biggest enemy to this day. I work out of my home. Sometimes I misplace things, and Kelly is witness to my irritability. He might not even know what I'm looking for, but when he hears me ranting he usually at least pretends he's helping me.

He makes me laugh, and my mood is better, and this almost always leads to a successful completion of my search.

One day, I couldn't find my telephone! The price of progress. Why, I remember the good old days when phones were attached to the wall. You didn't lose one then! I don't understand why people are so enamored with cordless phones! Why can't people leave well enough alone?

Okay, the previous paragraph is an example of one of my rants. Read it as if I were shouting. I could have written in all caps to signify loudness, but who likes that?

I didn't want you to read a book disproportionate with positives about me. I have my negatives. We're all human, after all. That's the tie that binds us.

Well, usually when I lose a phone, I push a button, and track down the beep. This time no beep could be heard. My frustration increased. Kelly couldn't find it either.

Fortunately, we have friends, and as our folk wisdom teaches, a friend in need is a friend indeed. We called Kathy Naretty and her husband, and told them we needed "fresh eyes." They came right over, and in a few minutes, found my phone.

Handling frustration—having good impulse control—is an essential component of parenthood. Parents can reinforce each other, when events put either one close to an edge.

The best advice we ever gave our children, as Kelly and I both believe, immediately preceded their respective marriages. We took each couple, for example, our daughter Paula and her future husband, out to dinner, just the four of us.

At an appropriate time, we told them, "We're going to give you one word of advice, and that's it." They looked at us with wide eyes. One word?

"You're going to have problems, and we don't want to hear about them."

I know, that's more than one word. It's one sentence. And we weren't finished.

"We think you will be able to solve your problems. Our main advice is, don't involve us. Don't involve friends. Don't involve anyone. Resolve your difficulties yourselves. That's the only advice we're going to give you."

Jimmy and Paula were kind enough not to volunteer a word or sentence count. Better still, they took our counsel to heart.

We had the same dinner with all five of our children and their soon-to-be mates, and gave the same advice, only with the last four we didn't use "one word" as a preface.

To this day, we have not heard any of our children complain to us about their spouse, just as our grandchildren don't complain about their cousins.

By the way, all my daughters used my wedding dress and veil, and my mother's waxed beaded crown. I appreciate the connection and earnestly hope my granddaughters continue the tradition.

Being a grandparent presents a whole new set of opportunities. Experience has taught the conscientious grandparent what works and what doesn't. The situation doesn't necessitate nearly as much discipline, and allows for creativity and play.

One afternoon Ruth's daughter, Kayla, was in our home playing. It was interesting to compare Kayla's play with that of her mother's when she was a child. So much energy!

Pretty soon, she asked for something to eat. My husband had purchased a bunch of fresh farm carrots, which he cleaned without removing the green, fluffy stems, and offered to Kayla, suggesting she hop around the yard.

Hop, hop, hop. That's what she did, holding her carrots, pretending to be a bunny.

Later, when it was Kayla's turn to bring a snack to school, she told Ruth that she wanted to bring carrots with "the fluffy stuff."

Another time, Sarah's daughter, Erin, was in her kindergarten class, and a classmate brought rice crispy cakes for everyone. Because it was St. Patrick's day, the cakes were dyed green. Erin told her teacher, "I can't eat that because it has food dyes in it."

You know, Erin was right. The parent ruined a healthy snack by putting green dye in it. I had talked to Erin about reading the label when you buy candy, and she heeded my advice.

When love is the foundation, advice does tend to stick.

I taught the children that one of the first steps toward financial health is to stay out of debt. Make your money work for you. Instead of borrowing to buy a new car, for example, save up for the purchase. If you do, it will cost you less.

I also tell them not to get into the credit card thing—never buy what you can't afford. To me, that is common sense. Or perhaps, in the modern "shop till you drop" mania, I might better describe it as "uncommon."

It's my good fortune that our children have never told Kelly and me, "Oh, you can't do this for your grandchildren because you're spoiling them." They've demonstrated the same trust in us that we have for them.

As for the grandchildren, I don't see them nearly enough.

Melina, Blake, and Michael live in Washington; Zachary and Alyssa live in California; Reece and Natalie live in Texas; Anna, Kayla, and Leah live in Indiana; and Erin, Molly, Bret, and Ryan live in Illinois.

Upon the birth of each grandchild, we open a brokerage account for her or his college education. We buy additional stock for their birthdays and for Christmas each year. I know my Dad would be proud of the family's financial progress, as well as its principles.

I send a note to each grandchild each year explaining the newest stock acquisition. It's pretty much the same letter every time, saying why we enjoy doing "nice" things for them, and listing everything about each of them that makes us proud.

I am frank with them because I respect them and trust in the respect they have for us. Our opinion matters! That's earned!

It's not that we're buying them. That is not the path to happiness. The Beatles were right: "Money can't buy me love."

Kelly and I are showing our grandchildren in different ways how much we admire and honor the kind of people they intend to be.

This doesn't mean we think they're never going to make mistakes. We understand mistakes, because we make our own.

We also stress the fact that when you are in high school, it's too early to decide who you are going to marry. So don't go steady.

Girls need to know a lot of different boys. Boys need to know a lot of different girls. That is far more important than being connected to just one as soon as possible.

We ask our children to tell their sons and daughters at the appropriate times: "You've had a couple of dates with the same person. Now he is going to have to date somebody else before he can date you again."

So now she has an excuse not to be tied to a person, who, at that age, probably only wants to control her.

I gave each grandchild a book on "How To Manage Your Savings." It's basically a primer—once one has a job—on how to save money by "paying yourself first," which is accomplished by putting a little bit into savings each month.

Grandparents can be teachers. But this is only possible within the boundaries of a happy relationship between grandparent and parent...a relationship built on love and (un)common sense.

One example—I could give 19—is my granddaughter Alyssa Sutton. Once, when she was visiting from California, she found my old baton and asked me to teach her how to twirl.

How exciting! For both of us!

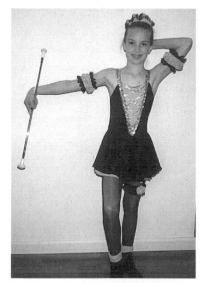
My baton twirler granddaughter

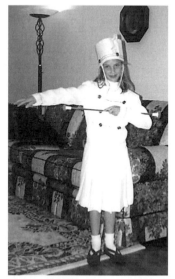
In her "Halloween costume"

Alyssa practiced so much that her arms were covered with black and blue marks. But she refused to quit, and continued to improve. Naturally, when it came time for her to return to her home in California, I gave her my baton.

In time she became more proficient than I had ever been. Her parents, Peter and Terri, arranged for baton lessons, and soon Alyssa competed in national contests, winning numerous awards.

Times do change, though. When I found my homemade majorette outfit in the attic and gave it to her, she used it for a Halloween costume.

Oh well!

I beg you to forgive my pride—shared by Kelly—at the handwritten messages on the anniversary cards sent to us in August of 2003.

From our daughter Ruth and her family: "Thanks for being so perfect!"

From our son Peter and his family: "You are the perfect example of what a marriage (and parents) should be."

I whole-heartedly wish every single (and married) one (or two) of you the happiness Kelly and I felt upon receiving these cards from our children.

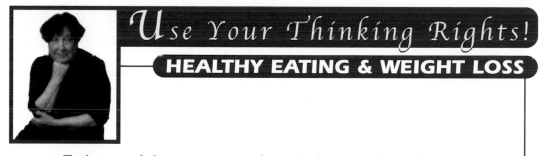

To lose weight, you must trim calories—total calories—no matter their source. I've said it before and I say it again (not for the last time):

"The only way to lose weight is to expend more calories than you eat."

Essentially, the most recent studies on weight loss diets confirm this old adage, proving that, whether it's high protein, high carbohydrate, or smartly balanced, a diet is really about calorie control.

The keys to decreasing your calorie intake are to eat healthy, eat smart, and eat less. The best method of increasing your calorie expenditure is to exercise.

Walking is an excellent choice. It is inexpensive, and the least likely to lead to injury. Did you know that walking a mile burns as many calories as running a mile?

We can chase our "ideal" weight like a greyhound pursuing a mechanical rabbit, but the smarter thing to do is to find a way to eat healthy and control calories, and then let the weight loss come naturally, as it will.

How can we make this happen? By using our thinking rights.

The IRS allows deductions for weight loss programs that are a part of the treatment for diseases such as obesity. Taxpayers who participate in these programs for medically valid reasons may be able to deduct amounts up to 7.5% of their adjusted gross income, similar to any other medical expenses not covered by insurance or other reimbursement.

Weight loss is not all vanity, but in the world as we presently know it, a preference for a pleasing physical profile possesses plenty of psychological power.

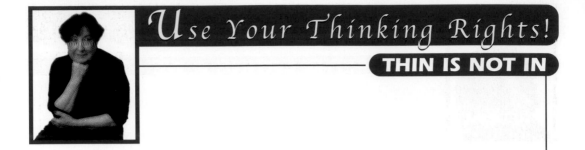

Thin claims to be "in," but I believe this is an unnatural and unhealthy goal. When I see someone really skinny, like many of the magazine models, I know they are not treating their body right.

Anyone consuming less than 1,200 calories per day may not satisfy the body's nutritional requirements. Most people eating more than 2,700 calories a day are going to gain weight.

Too little or too much. Two bad choices.

The right approach is to embrace a lifestyle where what you eat is what you need to keep your weight at a desirable level. Use your thinking rights.

Maintaining is just as good an idea as losing. Weigh yourself weekly, preferably the morning of the same day each week.

Some people are satisfied to be five to ten pounds overweight. Others approach the challenge of losing five pounds with the same fervor as an obese person determined to lose one hundred.

Our bodies are machines, and our food is fuel.

Put antifreeze in the gas tank, and the car won't run.

Take in too many calories, especially from unhealthy food, and sooner or later, the machine will malfunction.

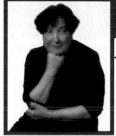

Cheat on your diet, and who are you cheating? Need I answer?

Don't worry. This type of cheating is not punishable by the certainty of failure. Every meal is a chance for a fresh start.

During the early stages of a diet, habits are being changed, and that's difficult. Cheating happens. Let's not become too angry with ourselves, or judge too harshly, in such challenging circumstances.

If you "eat wrong," feel free to grant—and accept—a self-pardon. Use your thinking rights. Don't permit yourself to become discouraged. As soon as possible, begin again.

Go forward a day at a time, with the intent and desire to strengthen your "eat right" willpower.

We are endeavoring to change our lifestyles. That can take time, so we must persevere.

It is incorrect to equate momentary setbacks with total failure. Name me a championship baseball team that went undefeated. Even the 1908 Cubs lost once in awhile.

The ideal is to eat right, maintain a desired weight, and, all the while, feel like we're eating the way we want, enjoying our food, and the entire dining experience.

Losing weight is a matter of making a choice.

Here's an example.

A woman who lost more than one hundred pounds on the Seattle Sutton's Healthy Eating program told me:

"After many false starts, one day I made a decision. I saw a picture of me taken at wedding reception, and I decided that's it, no more. I told myself, `being obese is not who I really am, and I will no longer accept it.`"

Consider the cornucopia of an American meal. The slab of meat, the pan of pie, the bowl of mashed potatoes. Milk, fruit, vegetables, bread, pudding, ice cream, gravy, and more, and more.

How much of this bounty should be consumed by someone dedicated to healthy eating and weight management? What portions should find your plate, and, ultimately, your mouth.

Less is usually enough. More is too much.

The steadily growing size of food portions is one of the causes of obesity in this country. Food manufacturers and the restaurant industry distort what the typical American believes is an appropriate amount to eat. Many people now perceive restaurant portions as the norm.

Likewise, when meals are served family style at home, the result is inadequate portion control. Meals should be served on individual plates. And portions should be sized with an eye toward calorie management.

If you become accustomed to a larger-than-necessary portion, well, maybe that's how you evaluate "being satisfied" with your meal. But you will be just as satisfied—and more likely to lose weight—with a smaller portion, once you get used to it.

Some food manufacturers have decided to sell smaller packages of cookies and other products, as a way to help the problem of obesity.

That's a good thing, for sure, but people need to remember it's not the number of cookies in the bag that really matters. It's easy to buy two bags. Or three!

Use your thinking rights. It's not the size of the container that counts. It's how many you put in your mouth.

Controlling the quantity of intake is ultimately up to the individual. Careful and intelligent meal preparation and portion management are an indispensable element of healthy eating.

By the way, that's what we do for our clients at Seattle Sutton's.

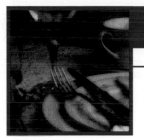

(MONDAY:)

Dinner: CHICKEN ALFREDO DINNER

Grilled seasoned chicken and medley of veggies drizzled with our low-fat
Alfredo sauce served on a bed of wild rice.

(TUESDAY:)

Breakfast: FRESH STRAWBERRY MUFFIN

And seasonal fruit.

Lunch: CHILLED POTATO, TURKEY FILLET AND FRESH VEGGIES

A beautiful display of roasted turkey, chilled cooked potato and other vegetables
ready for a dip in a tangy dill sauce.

Dinner: CHEESE LASAGNA

A blend of cheeses rolled in lasagna pasta, covered by an Italian style tomato sauce
along with tender Brussels sprouts and an orange cinnamon poached pear.

(WEDNESDAY:)

Breakfast: WHEAT BAGEL

With cream cheese and fruit juice.

Lunch: WHOLE BAKED POTATO WITH CHILI

The popular baked potato with ground turkey and vegetables in a tomato base
topped with aged Cheddar cheese.

Dinner: TETRAZZINI

Succulent pieces of meat, sliced mushrooms and linguini baked together
in a light sauce and topped with Parmesan cheese and paprika, served with
baked sweet potato and spiced apples.

(THURSDAY:)

Breakfast: SSHE'S ORIGINAL SLICED BREAKFAST BREAD

With fruited yogurt.

Lunch: CHICKEN SALAD WITH ANGEL FOOD CAKE

Tender morsels of white meat, fresh onion and celery pieces with
walnuts and raisins tossed in a flavorfully seasoned dressing along with a
Roma tomato, served with angel food cake.

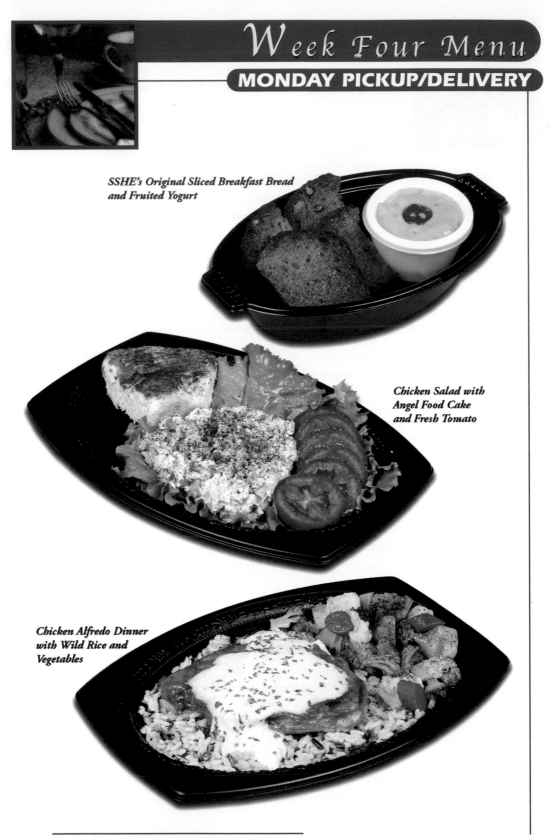

SSHE's Original Sliced Breakfast Bread and Fruited Yogurt

Chicken Salad with Angel Food Cake and Fresh Tomato

Chicken Alfredo Dinner with Wild Rice and Vegetables

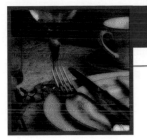

THURSDAY:

Dinner: HOMESTYLE MEATLOAF

A great tasting meatloaf made of turkey meat and seasonings topped with tomato sauce and served with garlic whipped potatoes, braised cabbage and cream style corn.

FRIDAY:

Breakfast: AUNT TILLIE'S BANANA MUFFIN
With fresh fruit.

Lunch: FAMOUS TUNA BUMSTEAD

A whole wheat English muffin topped with tuna and cheese, served with blue corn chips and fresh carrots.

Dinner: MANICOTTI

Manicotti noodles stuffed with Ricotta cheese smothered in an Italian style tomato sauce and sprinkled with aged Romano cheese, served with gourmet whole green beans.

SATURDAY:

Breakfast: FARM-FRESH CHEESE OMELET
With refreshing pineapple juice.

Lunch: MIXED GREEN SALAD

Mixed salad greens with chunks of cheese, croutons and creamy dressing, served with a fat-free chocolate brownie.

Dinner: CHICAGO STYLE CHILI

A good helping of pinto beans, onions, ground turkey and spices in a hearty tomato sauce with oyster crackers and Cheddar cheese for topping.

SUNDAY:

Breakfast: RAISIN BREAD
With tropical fruit.

Lunch: MACARONI & CHEESE

A favorite lunch of macaroni and robust cheese served with a colorful salad of sliced beets and onions.

Dinner: OVEN FRIED CHICKEN

Boneless chicken lightly coated with herbed bread crumbs, served with fresh squash, broccoli au gratin and a wheat dinner roll.

MONDAY:

Breakfast: CRANBERRY GRANOLA BAR
Fruit juice.

Lunch: ALL AMERICAN SANDWICH

Our homemade fruit spread and roasted peanut spread to use on fresh baked wheat bread slices, served with fresh fruit.

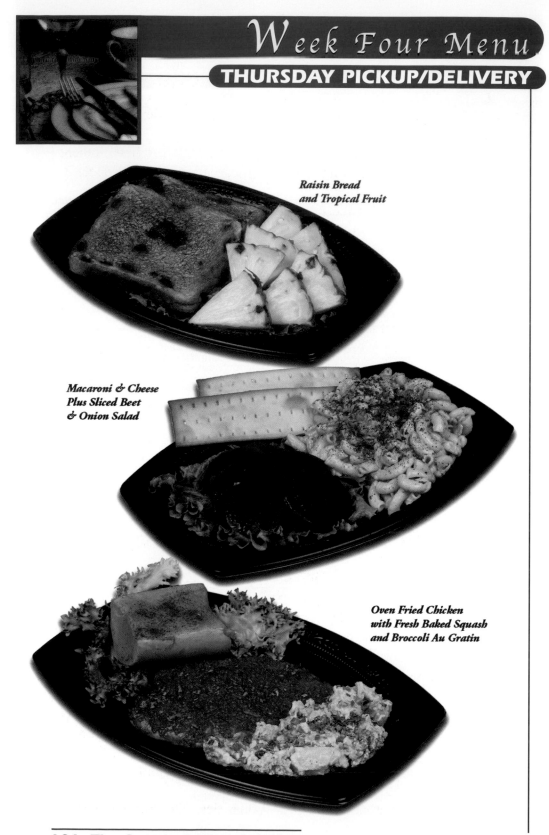

*Raisin Bread
and Tropical Fruit*

*Macaroni & Cheese
Plus Sliced Beet
& Onion Salad*

*Oven Fried Chicken
with Fresh Baked Squash
and Broccoli Au Gratin*

Chapter Nine

As time passed, my assistance in my husband's medical practice expanded to include giving weight loss, cholesterol lowering, and realistic diet instructions to our patients. We never charged for this service.

I did my best to help these people lose weight. The first element was (and is) communicating an overall understanding of the necessary strategy and tactics.

"Healthy eating" is the strategy, and "selecting and preparing the right foods" are the tactics.

The foundation of weight loss, as I've said before and will say many times again, never changes. Whether the time period in question is a day, a week, a month, or a year, weight is gained, maintained, or lost according to the body's flawless, automatic calculation of calorie intake vs. calorie expenditure.

Because of my nature, in general, and my concern for my father, in specific, I threw myself without barrier or hesitation into this aspect of Kelly's work, familiarizing myself with the science of healthy eating, reading articles and experiment summaries, asking questions, collecting as much data as possible.

It wasn't difficult to persuade patients to value better eating habits, nor did any of them have a problem evaluating the veracity of calories in vs. calories out. No overweight person I counseled suggested that gaining additional weight was the pathway to good health.

They were with me—in body and spirit—as we sat together examining the guidelines which would help them lose weight and gain health. But a stealth fear of failure undercut our conversations, undermining the patient's confidence—and mine.

Simply put, it is one thing to read the recommendations for losing weight and lowering cholesterol…and quite another to acquire ingredients, and prepare meals.

"Easier said than done" is more than a cliché. It's an accurate characterization of the human condition at this point in our psychological and spiritual development.

My frustration increased as one well meaning and well-motivated patient after another failed (despite consistently sincere and sometimes desperate attempts) to follow the guidelines.

Some, of course, were able to follow the menus, and this was good for them, and satisfying to Kelly and me.

Many of our patients were Type 2 diabetics. Dr. Sutton would instruct me to prepare a menu with a precisely calculated caloric exchange system. To do so was primarily our responsibility, because the nearby hospital at Ottawa had only one dietician, who was never in Marseilles.

I knew that what we were doing wasn't exactly meeting the needs of all our patients. Handing someone a sheet of paper isn't necessarily the right answer. But how could we improve?

Many of the people I was counseling, vexed by an inability to stick to a healthy eating plan, repeated a similar theme: "If someone would cook the meals, I would eat them."

I heard the words, but, as with most people when the future reaches back in time and addresses them, didn't realize the message was prophetic. The real meaning took a while to work itself into my mind.

Meanwhile, it became clear that we needed a bigger and more modern medical facility. By now, Kelly had a physician's assistant, Rod Full, working with him. Rod was excellent. With his help, we were treating more patients. That's one reason we needed more space.

In 1975, it became the responsibility of the three of us (Kelly, Rod, and I) to oversee the project. Our guiding principle: design and build a medical facility that would allow Dr. Sutton, Rod, and the patients to be very comfortable, and also permit the practice to flourish in an efficient and pleasant environment.

Since we still lived in the house Dr. Clark had helped us buy, I had never experienced the pleasure of creating a home. My role in designing and planning the new office filled my psychological need to create in a material way, and gave me experience in designing without a pattern.

Something in me—essential to my deepest sense of self-expression—vigorously responds to any creative challenge. No matter the project, I wake up in the middle of the night, thinking, "Oh my gosh, that's a good idea. What if I forget by the morning?"

I have learned to keep a notebook and pen on a bedside table, so I can scribble a little note as a reminder.

Kelly's office had to meet certain specific needs—office space, examination rooms, waiting room, etc. Given the fulfillment of these required utilitarian criteria, we made our facility as comfortable and pleasant as possible.

By the way, our sons Pete and Chris installed the electrical wiring in the building.

In 1979, my father succumbed to congestive heart disease. Too soon! Too soon! If only...

Things changed after my father's death. Soon the last of our children left the house for college. I was too busy to have the "empty nest" syndrome, but I did miss my children—my friends—every day. Not that we don't see each other quite a bit. But any additional time is always a plus.

We also look for opportunities to spend time with non-family friends. In December of 1983, a dozen of us—six couples—decided to share a vacation together in Las Vegas. Kelly and I checked in at the registration desk, and rode the elevator to our floor.

We didn't realize two people were stalking us. I guess the sanctuary of our life in Illinois made us less wary of danger in "routinely" safe circumstances. We didn't even consider the possibility that someone might push into our room and rob us.

We were wrong. These two—a man and a woman—entered, shut the door, and demanded our money. Kelly resisted. "No!" he said, and told me, "Scattle—yell!"

One of the robbers stood at the door. I couldn't open it, but I started screaming. He grabbed me around the neck, and tried to take my purse, draped over my shoulder. He couldn't.

The other robber—a woman—tried to stab Kelly with a darning needle. Everything happened so fast. I thought, "Is that a knife she has?"

We had our coats on—very warm in the room, and the struggle seemed to last longer than it probably actually did. We fought them while I continued to scream for help.

Kelly took the darning needle from his assailant, and suddenly—hallelujah—hotel security arrived on the scene. Our friends in the next room—the Bettassos—had heard our shouts and called for help.

Both robbers were subdued and arrested. They had criminal records, and were wanted by the law for other similar crimes.

We pressed charges and came back for their trial. Kelly and I felt this was important, even if inconvenient. We didn't want these criminals to escape justice, and attack other people.

During the hotel room fight, a bizarre thought flashed through my head, "Oh my goodness. If these people murder us so close to Christmas, our children will feel bad during the holidays."

I didn't want to ruin their Yule celebration. As if they'd feel better if we were killed in July.

About this time, liquid diets became the "in-thing." Their popularity—and that of Nutri-System—soon came to our attention.

People came into the office with slips of paper for him to sign "okaying" them to go on one liquid regime or another. Kelly refused.

"I don't have any idea what these so-called diets are all about," he said. "Where's the scientific evidence that they work and are healthy?"

The whole liquid diet ho-de-do raised the idea of healthy eating back to the forefront of my thoughts. I was still counseling obese patients, of course, and now I had to help them think through this new—and gimmicky—approach.

I quickly came to the conclusion that—like all fad diets— a liquid one might have short-term weight-loss effects. But the patient's real life eating habits were not affected. No liquid diet can last forever, and as soon as it ends, the "thinner" patient now tends to self-reward by gorging on solid food.

"I'm sacrificing now," is the gimmick diet mind-set, "I'll make up for it later." Trouble is, after he does, he's no longer "thinner."

By the way, if all humans chose the liquid diet route, how long before evolution, perceiving no need for teeth, removed them? That would change the idea of beauty in most cultures. Are you psychologically prepared for the "Ms. Toothless" pageant circa 2525?

Paula was the first of our daughters to get married. My first cousin, Alton Zenker, led the wedding prayers. Alton eventually became a Bishop in the Lutheran Church.

Paula's wedding reception was an old-fashioned German "hochzeit." That means: "Happy Time." It certainly was!

I taught the caterer how to make the German dish "Knepfla." This food, and the name, were invented in the Gackle area. Knepfla is an instant noodle, made by dumping pieces of dough into boiling water.

The best part for me was planning the festivities with Paula. I know that people get stressed out by pre-wedding necessities. My advice is to treasure the planning experience. Remember, it's the last time to plan something with your daughter before she's married and has family responsibilities of her own.

Planning together is quality time. Enjoy it! The wedding doesn't have to come out perfect. For example:

We had Paula's reception at our home, complete with a strolling violinist, Louis Nanni. However, Nanni, a Marseilles shoe cobbler with a real talent for music, stumbled on an electric cord during his performance, and cut his head.

Kelly, resplendent in his wedding tux, drove Nanni to the office five blocks away, sewed his wound with five stitches, and brought him back. He insisted on continuing to play. What a warrior!

Many out-of-town friends and relatives stayed at the homes of our friends in Marseilles. Years later, I'm still trying to catch up by offering our home, most recently for visitors attending a wake.

Ruth and Sarah had their own versions when it came time for their weddings. Both receptions were at our house. Ruth celebrated with a Polish theme, Sarah with a Swedish. The latter's wedding reception was called a "brollop," Swedish for "happy time." Ruth's party was called a "przyjmowanie," which means "Polish party." It's a small world, as the song goes, after all.

Wise folk say that true genius has the capacity to perceive the ordinary in an extraordinary way. Sometimes it's not genius at all, it's the idea trying to work it's way into the world.

That's why I don't think it's right to take credit for what happened when Rodney Juergensen came into the office in 1985. Rodney is a Type 2 diabetic who needed to lose weight. My husband told me how many calories to allot him daily, and I put together a menu that did just that.

Like so many times before, I had a frustrated feeling that words on paper would not get translated into food on plate. I sighed, and Rodney sighed. Both of us knew we were participating in a futile exercise. So sad!

At that moment, the universe, having been unable to get me to grasp the right idea so many times before, refined its suggestive technique. Rodney spoke a familiar sentence, but he added his own distinctive twist.

"I'm not going to do all that work," Rodney admitted. Instead of adding, "Not to say I wouldn't be able to follow this diet if someone prepared the meals," he told me, "I'd follow this diet if you prepared the meals."

One little word—"you." The gate opened. It wasn't narrow at all. In fact, it was wide enough to let in the future for which I had been preparing all my life.

My thoughts flashed: "How honest of him. Hmmm, I know a lot of patients that could do really well if they had someone prepare their meals. How could I make this happen?" Possible answers were in my mind as I asked the questions.

In a flash, I visualized the entire concept—so fast and yet so thorough. I knew the decisions I would have to make—and the information I would need. I saw the pitfalls—and the possibilities. In a bright instant. Every aspect.

How can I take credit? I didn't summon the idea, though I was delighted by its arrival. My future, courtesy of Rodney Juergensen, brought itself to my attention.

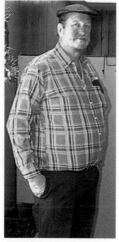
Rodney Juergesen

That afternoon I talked with Kelly about the thoughts that Rodney had prompted. Did the good doctor think a healthy meal preparation service would truly benefit his patients?

"Yes," began his answer. "Probably," he concluded.

My respect for his judgment—and caution—brought me to a crossroads. Which path would I take?

Did I want to start a new business? From scratch? After all, I was 53 years old. And busy. Did I have the energy? Yes, as mentioned, I've been blessed with an energy surplus. Did I have the desire? Theoretically.

I pondered the choice. I've always been a person who needed a challenge. The kids were out of the house and raising their own families, so that left an opening. The medical practice was organized and humming along. Our clinic was complete and functioning as intended. I could remain content with assisting Kelly.

Anyway, I had earned the right to rest if I desired, after working hard for so many years. Money was no longer a major concern.

Did I want to coast for the rest of my life? Not that there's anything wrong with that. Or did I want to take my experience and maturity into a new project, which I honestly felt would benefit many?

I chose nursing as a career to comfort the sick and assist the healing process. I raised my children to be happy in the world. Was developing a healthy eating program consistent with my basic values for self-expression? Was it worth the time and trouble? Would I be happy?

Yes, yes, yes!

I told Kelly my decision, and reassured him that I wouldn't quit helping him at the clinic. He was relieved to hear that, I know, and very supportive.

That night I tried to slow my mind, and outline a plan in writing. The process had many similarities to the design of the medical clinic.

I knew the desired result, and the requirements, and had an overall plan. Now I needed to make sure the individual problem-solving elements worked in single, and combination.

If I were going to make meals, they would have to be as healthy as possible. Every step of the process had to be done the right way. The pure way. The fair way. Eliminate any necessity for people to plan, shop, cook, and portion.

Three meals a day. Seven days a week. Calories carefully counted and calculated. Guaranteed to meet the basic nutritional needs of any person, regardless of age, sex, weight, or general state of health.

I knew that if I made it possible for people to eat what they should, they would feel better about themselves, and this attitude would help them in their daily lives. That's the ticket.

No gimmicks. No tricks. No contracts.

People could purchase their meals a week at a time. If they desired to stay with the program, they could keep buying. If not, they would be free to go…and come back later, if they wanted.

My diet had to be constructed on a base of science and common sense. My program would merit the approval of knowledgeable doctors and dieticians.

Meals had to be served fresh, and include salads and fresh fruit.

A first-class preparation and delivery system would have to be devised, involving professional kitchens and refrigerated trucks.

No harmful additives could be part of the meals, no artificial sweeteners, no MSG, no food dyes.

The whole plan revolved around observations I had been making for decades. Many people do not want to spend—or do not have—kitchen time. Yet they want to eat healthy.

Meeting that need was—and is—the essence of my vision.

I had to guide my diet into the real world by building a business and staying true to my plan. Starting any business is risky. Starting a brand new company providing a brand new service—never done before—might be almost impossible.

Great! A worthwhile challenge! Batter up!

I understand the value of caution. But, in the words of Albert Einstein, "I'd rather be an optimist and wrong than a pessimist and right."

An excellent philosophy—especially when you're using your own money. I set aside $1,000 to develop the company, and threw myself into the project, after promising Kelly that I wouldn't let it interfere with my work in his clinic.

That meant I had to work in my spare time. Many a night I stayed up late, examining components, honoring the counsel of Lao Tzu, as quoted in Chapter One, and Rene Descartes, who articulated the same concept like this: "Solve a big problem by breaking it into a whole bunch of little ones."

Even after I fell asleep, my thinking did not stop. Like so many times previously, I woke and made notes.

One Saturday afternoon Kelly drove me to Eldorado to visit his family. All the way—600 miles round trip—I peppered him with questions. He was so patient! And his advice, as always, helped me focus on the real issues. I took notes on his answers, and scribbled my own thoughts.

No matter where I found myself, if I had a speck of free time, I turned it into a "Healthy Eating" moment. I studied, thought, and wrote constantly.

Organizing the business. Planning the first menus. Tracking every conceivable detail. I've never taken a course in French, but my grandchildren say that when you study a language that you appreciate, you're constantly living it and thinking it, even when you're not speaking it. That's what the early days were like. Talk about being in a zone!

On the first day, I wrote down two basics around which I would build my company. No matter what happened, I pledged to myself, I would never deviate from either. Here they are: "Customer needs have first priority," and "Deliver on all promises."

Starting with my friends, I spread the word. Kathy and Dick Naretty invited Kelly and me to a backyard party. Their other guests remember that I joined the fun with a copy of the Wall Street Journal under my arm.

A headline blared: "Out of the Kitchen in the New Millennium."

The story it heralded theorized that by early in the 21st century American kitchens would contain only a microwave and a refrigerator. Stoves and ovens would be extinct.

Per the headline, the story reported that, by the turn of the century, people would not spend much time in their kitchen except to use their refrigerator and microwave.

"This is the key to my new idea," I told the party guests. They were all a little worried about me, as I later discovered, but, being friends, were supportive and encouraging. They did point out that I knew "nothing" about the food industry.

I agreed, but assured them that wasn't going to stop me. I have never been afraid to ask questions and honestly evaluate the meaning of the answers. How else can we learn?

Why would anyone have faith that a small-town nurse with no previous experience could build a groundbreaking business? Well, I believed. So did Kelly. That's enough confidence to make a good start, and earn the opportunity to keep progressing.

Chapter Ten

Onward!
Slowly. With no model to follow. But surely, regardless. Some days the enormity of the project overwhelmed me. Could we possibly succeed? I fought my apprehensions and kept moving forward, because I knew I was working to create something people needed and would appreciate.

Anyway, as previously revealed, I am an optimist. Even before we served our first meals, I believed the business would grow rapidly and expand quickly. That's the state of mind I bring to the table (no pun consciously intended, although I happily acknowledge the serendipity).

My planning relied on common sense, which I define as the mental and physical application of everything a person has learned. Ideas extend from the mind first in thought, then design, and, finally, action.

I mentally sorted every aspect of the idea, determined to create a system built on the best thinking of which I am capable. The challenge may appear daunting. So much to plan! So much to do!

Good work should follow a few simple guidelines:

Keep organized. Proceed by doing. Don't postpone unnecessarily. Use all your skills. Focus on the overall goal, as well as the task at hand.

Think through the options. Analyze the specific objectives that need to be met. Then, everything considered, mental, emotional, and conscience, do what feels right.

Don't be a person who is afraid of making mistakes. I believe in making my choices, taking my actions, and not feeling bad about criticism.

My advice to others is the same as my advice to myself. "If you do what you know is right, you shouldn't worry about what anybody says." In the end, when things work out, your critics will say, "Oh, she knew what she was doing."

If they don't recognize the facts, that's their problem.

Conversely, if the second-guessers turn out to be right, it's my duty to acknowledge that. If I don't, that's my problem. So what? I'm not afraid of being wrong. I like to learn.

Following your best sense of what to do is a sure-fire way to be happy. Happiness is good.

When bad things happen, I've always been one to think, "Things will get better." I hope. I expect. I keep trying. If I didn't, I might become depressed. That's not my choice.

I spent weeks designing an appetizing and healthy menu. At the beginning, I couldn't promise much variation. There were only a few meals in the rotation.

I gave thorough attention to every detail. I didn't want to be bluffing when I claimed our meals were healthy. I wanted to be sure we were implementing the best of medicine and food science.

To make sure my food choices were healthy, I called Mahmood Kahn (PHD, RD), an associate professor of Food Service Management at the University of Illinois, and outlined my idea.

He listened patiently, asked a lot of questions, and, after due consideration, gave me his support. He thought we were taking the "correct approach" and would benefit our clients.

Subsequently, Dr. Kahn became a food analysis consultant to the company. His students conducted the first tests of my meals. Our recipes and ingredients are now—and always have been—researched, analyzed, tested, and re-tested.

Why? Our menu planning, food selection, preparation, and delivery must be consistent with the most rigorous standards. The only way to be sure is to test.

The opposite approach—which I obviously disdain—is to rely on surveys to evaluate people's reactions, and then change the menu accordingly. Well, political polling is an insidious enemy of a strong democracy, and marketing surveys pose the same threat to healthy eating.

Polling makes politicians good at manipulating public opinion instead of providing genuine leadership and creative problem solving. Surveys are a poor substitute for quality thought and creative intuition.

From early on, so-called marketing experts urged me to poll my customers, and alter my menus accordingly. I always refused. I did not see the value of asking my customers, who were counting on me to give them healthy meals, "What don't you like?"

Because I'm determined to serve people the food they should eat, I won't sacrifice quality for popularity, even if it increases sales. Which I doubt anyway. When people get tired of gimmicks and failure, they're ready for us. All we have to do is let them know who and where we are.

My husband and I are on the meal plan, and that's a big help when it comes to adjusting the menu.

Marketing consultants seemed to spring out from behind the bushes. With polished presentations and gleaming eyes, they urged me to "use the latest techniques." Sometimes I felt as if they were predators and I was prey.

They had "modern ideas" for me to use, like giving people menu choices, or selling less than 21 meals per week. It's important to listen, and some of their presentations seemed reasonable, but my style is to think ideas through to their consequences. I don't find it wise to budge from my goal of improving "eating habits."

With Dr. Kahn's participation verifying the meal's health benefits, I felt I had built the necessary foundation. I named the company "Diet-Carry-Out," formed a corporation, hired three people, and rented space from a local caterer in Marseilles.

I was determined to find loyal and trustworthy employees. I knew I would be good to them, and I expected the same in return. If they didn't reciprocate the feeling, well, frankly, I didn't want their help.

To achieve this goal, I veered from the normal course and decided not to place an ad in the paper. Instead, I relied upon my husband, who knew almost everyone in Marseilles. He had been in their homes, seen them under stress, and has a very good feel for stability and character.

Because I spent a full workday at the clinic before reporting to Diet-Carry-Out, and was not physically present during normal working hours, how could I know who was likely to carry out assignments in the right way, and who was not?

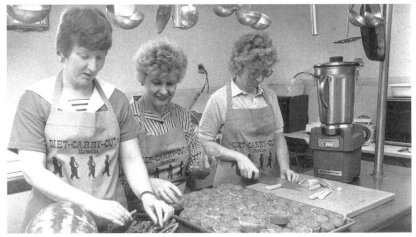

Three of our early employees Sal Clark,
Carol Macchietto, Pat Kesler

"Kelly," I asked, "Do you think (so-and-so) would do well as an employee of mine?" And he would give me his considered opinion. He was always right.

Many of my friends recommended that I ask Rosemary Martin to be my first employee and manager. Rosemary turned out to have an energetic, vivacious personality. She accepted the job and helped launch the company. We became fast friends.

The first employees did turn out to be exceptionally loyal and hard-working. Plus we had a lot of fun. Without these wonderful people, I am sure we wouldn't be where we are today.

We officially started serving meals September, 15, 1985. I selected the name Diet-Carry-Out, because I wanted people to know exactly what we did—provide a diet that customers could pick up or have delivered. It wasn't that good of a name—too generic—but I liked it at the time.

We grew slowly and carefully because we still had so much to learn. Development of the menus, food analysis, labeling, longer distance delivery, a distributor system—structuring the whole business actually—needed time.

Most of the initial customers were my friends from church, or my husband's patients. Rodney Juergensen was one, of course.

We served 231 meals our first week. Eleven customers!

Our meal preparation procedure dedicated two days a week for prepping and baking, two days for cooking and packaging, and two days for delivery and pick-up. We used to joke that we were the Henry Ford of meal preparation assembly lines.

We prepared the meals in space leased from the local Marseilles caterer. That's where I showed up early most mornings. Because my morning time at Diet-Carry-Out was limited, I sometimes rose from bed at 4:30 a.m. to go there, and help put the turkeys in oven, etc. My main task was to organize the day's work. I also did whatever housekeeping needed doing, including washing pots and pans.

Kelly's physician's assistant started seeing patients at 8 a.m., so I opened the medical clinic by then. Rod could help some people, but the more serious cases waited to see Kelly when he got back from his morning hospital duties, making rounds and occasionally assisting in surgery.

During the day, I managed the business aspect of the clinic, per usual, and brought Diet-Carry-Out lunch for Dr. Sutton and his physician's assistant. Their work-load was too heavy to allow them to leave the clinic. My duties didn't end until 5 p.m. (sometimes later).

We put in a special telephone line at the clinic for Diet-Carry-Out business. Calls came frequently. Good. I loved to hear that telephone ring.

When my "day job" was done, I returned to the caterer's building, and tried to get a read on how things were going. I helped wherever necessary, often with the packaging. Finally, when we had finished the work at hand, I used the rest of the evening planning our growth.

My age turned out to be an advantage. Taking on an entrepreneurial challenge of this nature while younger would have been impossible. The children! I could not have done this if they were still at home.

In the beginning, we only had a nine-day menu rotation. I had never been involved with institutional cooking. It had made sense to divide the work logically. This gave us the anchor of a "Here's What We Do Today" schedule, helping us move forward, and serving as a base for our fledgling business.

We still follow the same general procedures, though we're much more detailed now. We've learned a lot. Just like Ford.

Many a day I found comfort in an unpretentious and mundane routine. "Well, we have to wash the dishes (or bake the muffins) before we can do anything else." We were auto-didactic, continually tinkering with our procedures, learning on the job.

Working on the chores at hand also helped me understand the practical challenges we were certain to face in the future. How would we eventually make deliveries to Chicago, and other cities and states?

It's an exciting on-the-edge feeling to be moving forward successfully, while at the same time having so much to learn. I didn't know, for instance, that food could be measured with ladles.

No one, in my opinion, can survive the pitfalls of such a daring journey without an absolute willingness to make dispassionate observations, and prudent adjustments. Read and react! Learn and thrive!

Too little ego…nothing ventured.

Too much ego…nothing gained.

In the ensuing years, I always attended the Illinois Dietetic Convention. Our company would purchase a booth. Many dieticians stopped by—more every year—to learn more about Diet-Carry-Out. They are supportive!

"What a good idea!" Yes, we heard this again and again. Dieticians praised our food and our system. Most of all, as time went by, they reported that their patients did well on our meals.

Every year I returned from that convention in a happy cloud.

"Euphoric" is the most accurate adjective I can use.

Positive feedback is always helpful. When it comes from professionals in your field, it takes on added importance.

My belief in the benefits of our program didn't need much reinforcement. Nevertheless, I considered the source, and I cherished the affirmation. You can be confident, and still enjoy the lift of being praised by people you trust.

Meanwhile, back in the competitive world, we were slowly increasing our expertise, and winning new clients and supporters.

The Ottawa Daily Times, always supportive of Diet-Carry-Out, printed many articles about us, all favorable. One promoted the belief that the company would end up serving meals all over the nation, because "Seattle Sutton is giving people superior meals, like everybody's great-grandmother used to cook."

Noting this publicity, and wondering how it would affect Kelly's patients, my husband and I agreed that we would make sure that none of them ever felt obligated to order the meals. We decided never to talk about the business unless a patient asked. Then, and only then, Kelly would have me explain Diet-Carry-Out, and give them a choice.

In 1986, the Marseilles Chamber of Commerce named me "Boss of the Year." The Daily Times said I was chosen because I had a "super sense of humor," and was able to "laugh at my mistakes." Maybe that's because I had so much practice.

I like this quote the Daily Times had from one of my employees, whom they did not identify: "Seattle is a boss, a leader, a listener, a friend, and, best of all, a co-worker. Most bosses are 'bossy,' but not Seattle."

Please forgive my boldness in including this quote. I value it, and realize that a good boss requires good employees, and vice versa.

In the beginning, I took no salary, and placed no profit in my pocket, because I thought any money remaining after the expenses of preparing and delivering the meals should be used to build the company.

It wasn't a difficult decision. Most people who start a business have to take money out of it just to live. Let's face it. I was blessed. Kelly had become a very successful doctor. We had our own clinic.

My business financial challenge was to meet the payroll and pay all my bills. I can't sleep at night if my bills aren't promptly paid. That's the way I was raised. Almost always, the day we get a bill is the day we pay that bill. It's that important to me.

I have a policy that if any distributor doesn't pay their bills on time and we are notified at headquarters, we put that distributor on notice that they have no more than two days to settle the debt.

Bad credit affects all distributors. I won't have that. We're in business. Our suppliers are in business.

Other distributors appreciate our stance. It's as simple as this:

You have a right to expect your invoices to be paid in a timely manner, and you have a duty to pay your bills by their due date.

Our customers pay us before we make their meals. Why? Because I want to stay in business.

We order our ingredients based on our orders. Our meals are always served fresh, and, from the beginning, we have always done our best to keep the price low. If we allowed a situation where some people would cancel, we wouldn't survive. Food waste! Price increase!

That wouldn't be fair to the 99% of our customers who wouldn't dream of harming the company. As much as I believe in trust, I'm not naïve. I know there's always maybe one per cent that would like to take advantage. That's why you have to have—and must follow—strict and fair policies.

Fair, yes, to all, and beneficial to those with good intentions.

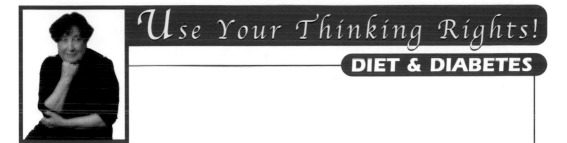
It's too bad that the two different diseases known as Type 1 and Type 2 are both labeled as diabetes.

A Type I diabetic is a true diabetic. This disease is usually inherited and causes the pancreas to malfunction its production of insulin.

The primary causes of Type 2 diabetes are nutrition and lifestyle choices. Genetics may play a role.

Up to eighty per cent of Type 2 diabetics are obese. Though the pancreas produces insulin, the body reaches a size which can't be adequately serviced, and the cells are unable to respond to whatever insulin is provided.

In other words, a pancreas that generates sufficient insulin for an 180-pound body may not meet the requirements of 280-pounder. Consequently, most Type 2 diabetics can benefit from weight loss.

Healthy eating cannot make the Type 1 pancreas produce insulin, but it can reduce body weight and this can be very helpful for Type 2 diabetics.

When the Type 2 diabetic loses weight, insulin resistance is lowered, thus allowing natural insulin to do a better job at lowering blood glucose levels, and providing a real possibility of a reduction or elimination of diabetes medication. I have seen this many times with people on Seattle Sutton's Healthy Eating regime.

Weight reduction also improves blood fat levels and blood pressure. All in all, there's no question we need to promote healthy eating and weight loss as a sound treatment for most Type 2 diabetics. We also should strive to stop ourselves, our families and our friends from gaining excess weight in the first place.

Treatment of diabetes costs approximately $100 billion every year. A healthy diet has many benefits!

If you're an overweight Type 2 diabetic, or fear you might become one, use your thinking rights.

Eat smart! Eat healthy!
Lose weight! Get well!

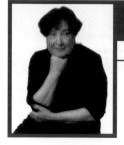

Obesity related diseases are the second-leading causes of premature loss of life—behind smoking—and are implicated in 300,000 deaths yearly. Furthermore, the rate of obesity has increased nearly 10% in the last decade.

I don't see the point of being diplomatic about such a life and death choice. People have to escape from the cycle of mindless habit and relentless denial.

Do you want to live? Or do you want to die?

If your in-the-heart answer is "live," then eating right is an absolute necessity. Eat healthy, and you are less likely to develop cardiac disease and coronary obstruction. If your diet is unhealthy, you are likely to become overweight or obese, and this often leads to congestive heart failure and hypertension.

After years of hypertension, twice as common in the obese, the heart eventually enlarges, becomes strained, and loses the ability to function properly.

A study of 5,881 men and women published in New England Journal of Medicine showed the risk of heart failure is double in obese people, and 34% higher in those categorized as "overweight."

Another study concluded that losing weight could prevent one of every six cancer deaths in the United States. Excess weight contributes to cancers of the breast, uterus, colon and rectum, kidneys, esophagus, gall bladder, cervix and ovaries, multiple myeloma, non-Hodgkin's lymphoma, pancreas, liver, and in men, prostate.

Anytime someone develops cancer of any kind, if they have eaten properly—and continue (or begin) to do so—they can more readily resist the disease and tolerate chemotherapy. A weight gain of just eleven pounds can double the risk of developing Type 2 diabetes.

In yet another study, researchers have found a striking relationship between being overweight at age 70 and developing Alzheimer's.

I ask you again. Do you want to live?

Do you want good health?

If your answer is yes, use your thinking rights. Find a way!

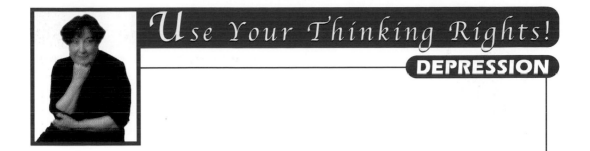

In some instances, the medical profession and the rest of us make a basic mistake in the diagnosis of depression. True, the diagnosis may be technically accurate, but we don't fully understand a potential source.

Many times the answer is right before our eyes. On occasion, depression is caused by the simple fact that the person in question—maybe our best friend—is carrying too much weight.

Even when it isn't clinical, being overweight can cause people to become defensive and over-protective. Perhaps they are contrasting their body with those of television stars and magazine models.

Their "better" self is harder to express, because the excess poundage has undermined their self-image and self-confidence.

Health problems associated with being overweight are an added burden.

Regaining self-esteem and self-confidence are vital to recovery. In some cases, instead of medicating this kind of depressed person, we should be helping them find a way to lose weight. Pills may only treat the symptom, not the cause.

Healthy eating, calorie control, and portion management are the keys to permanent weight loss. True for one and all, whether happy or depressed.

If depression continues after weight loss, well, that is a different situation, and may require additional treatment.

But in most cases, weight loss improves, if not restores, self-esteem, and this opens the door to a happier future.

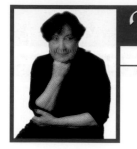
Sometimes it takes a crisis to make a family realize the importance of healthy eating. One example is the aftermath of a non-fatal heart attack.

The family must muster their total resources to meet the physical and emotional requirements of helping the patient recover. Many elements are involved, but let's focus on healthy eating.

Possibly, the heart attack itself has been brought on by unhealthy eating habits. No matter what previous efforts have or have not been made, the challenge-at-hand is stark and undeniable.

Eat healthy and live well.

But how can a family change a lifetime of bad eating habits?

Can meal choices be altered and improved so that the loved one can get better, and stay better? Yes.

Actually this difficult moment can be viewed as an excellent opportunity for a "food lifestyle change." Everyone involved can benefit.

For example, when a father has a heart attack as a result of years of unhealthy eating, a wise son will look in the mirror and see his own future, if his eating habits don't improve.

I actually think this is an instance in which a meal replacement approach is quite beneficial. This reduces stress and gives everyone more time with the loved one. Just make sure to find a company that guarantees healthy meals, and removes the worries of planning, shopping, and cooking.

Naturally I recommend Seattle Sutton's Healthy Eating. That's because I'm using my thinking rights.

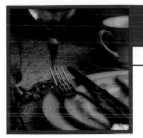
(MONDAY:)

Dinner: POLISH PIEROGIES WITH SAUSAGE AND SAUERKRAUT

Savory meal with ethnic overtones consisting of sausage, in-house sodium restricted sauerkraut, pierogies with a flavorful sauce, and sliced apples in plum sauce.

(TUESDAY:)

Breakfast: FRUIT SMOOTHIE DRINK

With apple-cinnamon muffin.

Lunch: ROBUST POTATO SKINS

A lunch favorite. Potato skins, cheese and a sour cream topping.
Served with fruit and dessert.

Dinner: FRENCH CREPE DINNER

A delicate creation of a chicken filled crepe beautifully displayed with
herb roasted Roma tomato and steamed green vegetable,
offered with succulent red raspberry delight.

(WEDNESDAY:)

Breakfast: MOIST & FLAVORFUL ORANGE BREAD

With cream cheese & fruit.

Lunch: FRESH SPRING SALAD

A heavenly salad with raspberry vinaigrette dressing, mandarin oranges,
and tender grilled chicken slices, served with a chilled vegetable
sipper and well seasoned flatbread cracker.

Dinner: MOSTACCIOLI

A cheesy Italian SSHE specialty of al dente pasta lightly covered with tomato sauce,
especially tasty with a healthy vegetable blend and a sundried tomato hardroll.
A heavenly salad with raspberry vinaigrette dressing, mandarin oranges,

(THURSDAY:)

Breakfast: ITALIAN STYLE FRITTATA

With fruit drink.

Lunch: TOMATO RICE STEW

A hearty tomato stew with crunchy whole grain cheese croustades.

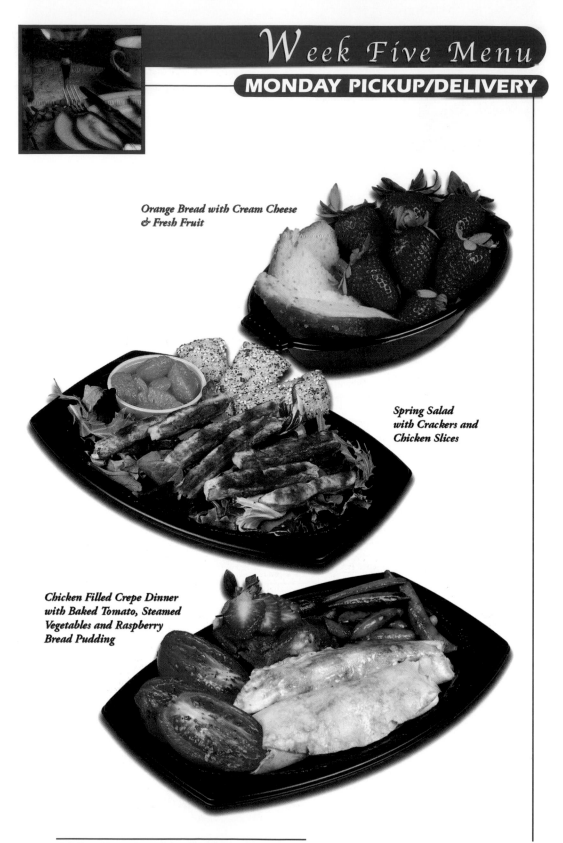

Orange Bread with Cream Cheese & Fresh Fruit

Spring Salad with Crackers and Chicken Slices

Chicken Filled Crepe Dinner with Baked Tomato, Steamed Vegetables and Raspberry Bread Pudding

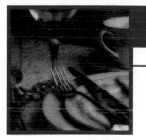

THURSDAY:
Dinner: ELEGANT CORNISH HEN
Oven roasted Cornish Hen with a delicate orange glaze, served with wild rice and a side of select baby beets and refreshing cranberry relish.

FRIDAY:
Breakfast: GRANDMA HELEN'S DELICIOUS CRANBERRY MUFFIN
With fresh fruit.
Lunch: FRESH CAESAR SALAD
Hearts of tender Romaine, Caesar dressing, and shredded cheese
served with a zucchini muffin.
Dinner: TUNA VEGGIE DELUXE DINNER SANDWICH
A delicious dinner sandwich on a sesame seed bun with tartar sauce, served with a delightful broccoli slaw tossed in an Oriental sesame dressing.

SATURDAY:
Breakfast: COUNTRY OMELET BREAKFAST
Petite omelet, breakfast sausage, juice and cinnamon swirl bread.
Lunch: POPULAR SPINACH CALZONE
A pocket filled with spinach, cheese and spices with a zesty sauce for dipping and a very tasty antipasto salad Italia for everyone to enjoy.
Dinner: CLASSIC STUFFED PEPPER
A fresh green pepper stuffed with seasoned rice and meat then baked just right accompanied by homestyle cornbread.

SUNDAY:
Breakfast: EILEEN'S FAVORITE FAMILY SECRET FRUIT BREAD
And citrus fruit.
Lunch: SOUTHWESTERN BEAN & PASTA SALAD
A tasty pasta salad with flavors of the southwest, plus a
delectable treat of Pacific pineapple bread pudding.
Dinner: ACAPULCO TACO PIE WITH CRUNCHY CORN SALAD
A wonderfully interesting combination of ground turkey, cheese and spices baked together along with avocado corn chips, authentic salsa, and a crunchy corn salad.

MONDAY:
Breakfast: WONDERFULLY FRUITY GERMAN GVACHA PASTRY
And apple juice.
Lunch: BBQ ON TEXAS CRUST
Meaty BBQ with shredded cheese atop a tasty crust, served with crisp garden fresh carrots and grapes.

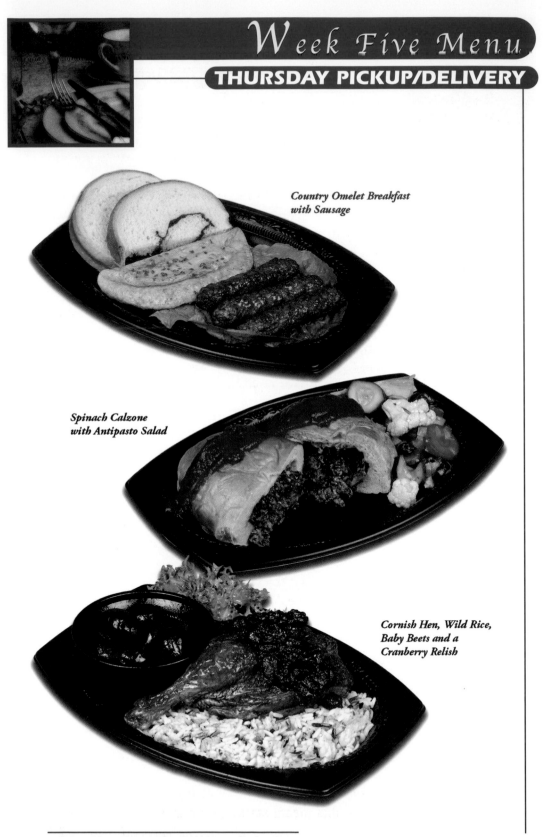

Country Omelet Breakfast with Sausage

Spinach Calzone with Antipasto Salad

Cornish Hen, Wild Rice, Baby Beets and a Cranberry Relish

Chapter Eleven

I think that almost all creative people like it when their ideas add happiness to the "mix." I know I do. The further an idea reaches into the world, the more people it involves and touches.

Why not design a project so that the better virtues of love and compassion are encouraged, instead of the baser ones of greed and selfishness?

To build the business, I followed two basic precepts. First, invest in marketing. Second, be exceptionally good to my loyal employees. I made sure to do plenty of both before I ever gave myself a salary.

Most of our profit dollars were thrown into the advertising budget. At first, all we could afford were late-night radio and television commercials in Chicago.

I used to set my alarm clock for when the ads were going to run, because I answered the 800 line.

Yours truly also appeared in the commercials. Even if more money had been available, I wouldn't have hired a professional announcer. Doing ours gave me the chance to tell listeners our story…in a factual and personal way.

I had several 800 lines installed in the house. Back then, we had no voice mail. I had to hustle when the phones started ringing.

If I knew a commercial was running at 2 a.m., I set my alarm so I would be ready. Kelly used to worry about me running through the living room in the middle of the night.

But I didn't want to miss even one call. I knew they were very important, and the ads were costly. It would be silly to blow the payoff, no matter the sacrifice in sleep.

By talking to potential customers, I got a feel for their honest reactions, and measured responses on a one-to-one basis. Much more satisfying—and valuable—than polling.

Frequently the calls concerned recovering heart attack patients still in their hospital beds. Either they or their relatives had been handed a low cholesterol, low fat diet. Having survived the original heart attack, they were now worried about following a diet that could help prevent another.

A comment I often heard from callers: "I have to take him home tomorrow, and how am I going to deal with his new food requirements?"

The very best way to commence healthy eating is to begin immediately. For the patients, this meant starting on our program as soon as possible. Then family members can spend their time taking care of their loved one and not worrying about planning, shopping, cooking, measuring, and cleaning up.

Virtually every caller was surprised to be talking to the person for whom the business was named. It seemed natural to me. I had many long conversations.

Most seemed grateful for the personal attention, and for the program. Even during the non-hospital calls, I often heard, "When can I start?"

Many went even further. "This is a dream come true…something I've been hoping might happen. I've wanted to eat right, but I haven't. Now I will."

Sometimes they called back after a week or two on our plan.

More than a few said, "I've never eaten food like this, because I never thought something good for me would taste good. Now I find out it's delicious. Thanks."

One of the benefits of personally answering calls was the opportunity to explain the company and its programs to potential distributors. Many people, after going on the meals for a month or so, called back with interest in becoming more involved.

"You've really got something going here," was a typical comment. "I want to join." And we would go from there.

Some nights, waiting for the phone to ring, I fantasized my father calling, and me answering the phone, and finally being able to help him.

Although that didn't happen, the fact that so many people expressed their gratitude for the program reinforced my determination to overcome all obstacles.

Building a company isn't the same as watching a toddler's video. A happy ending is not guaranteed.

We had to weather a few very real storms. Sometimes their source was an unpleasant surprise.

The local caterer appeared to enjoy providing space in his building. We all liked him. He was very nice. Sometimes he would decide on his own to fix lunch for all the employees. We had fun and so did he.

The caterer grew to understand our business, and as our meal count increased, he began to pressure me to sign a lease. I knew I couldn't. It wouldn't be long before we needed more space than he could provide.

One weekend he needed assistance catering a huge company picnic. We all went to help him. We cut watermelon, and served his guests—did everything as necessary. He paid a few of us, and offered to pay me. But it wasn't necessary. "It was fun," I told him, and refused his money. He manifested his gratitude vocally, and I felt glad about our friendship.

Two days later, he nervously delivered a lawyer's letter to my door stating that I had to sign a contract with him, or be out of the facility within 30 days!

I had always told him, "If there is anything you're not happy with, and you want us out of here, let me know." But his method of "letting us know" didn't set well with me. Why would he act so uncharacteristically?

Color me stunned and depressed. What to do? Our company was young and soon to be homeless. Could we overcome this blow? Could we find a solution?

Any new business, like a baby zebra born in an African veldt, has to struggle to survive its initial phase, when it is vulnerable, inexperienced, and relatively powerless. It's a rite of passage.

The world in which we live may seem to be best described by phrases like "Survival of the fittest," "Look out for number one," "Alliances of self-interest," and "Trust no one," but that's not necessarily an accurate understanding of reality.

Everyone has a choice. Maybe there will always be a few wild ones roaming around, ready to pounce, steal, and even kill. They have to be regarded in wisdom, and defended against with practical methods.

Too many folks are afraid that this is the only way of the world. Such a fear imprisons all who surrender to its tentacles. They are trapped by their own perception of a dog eat dog world. I don't choose to live there, so I didn't stay down long.

An opportunity presented itself. My husband's first office had been turned into a family house, and the tenants had just moved out.

Our close friends, Harold and Helen Danelson, joined me in assessing the place's food preparation possibilities. The Danelsons once had owned their own catering business, so they were familiar with what had to be done to satisfy all relevant ordinances.

They gave us their recommendations. It appeared as if we could turn this place into our new headquarters. Once again…a solution out of nowhere.

We cleaned and painted, had the carpeting taken out, new floors put in, and walls remade. Upstairs was designated as storage for packaging, dry goods, office supplies, and the like. Downstairs was for food preparation, though we still had a lot of equipment to purchase.

Harold Danelson knew of used restaurant equipment places in La Grange—Pierce Restaurant Equipment—and another in Peoria—La Hood. We still do business with both of them to this day.

Harold and I arrived at Pierce one morning in a huge van borrowed from Rod Full, and purchased enough equipment to completely fill it.

By the end of the day, that truck was flat-out crammed with ovens, coolers, worktables, and many other food preparation devices. I was particularly fascinated by Pierce's demonstration of the "Buffalo," a food chopper unlike anything I had ever seen. Harold assured me, "That's what you need."

He and I drove the borrowed and stuffed rig back to Marseilles. The temperature outside reached 100 degrees. Our vehicle had no air conditioning, so we kept cool by drinking ice water.

When we reached my driveway, several of our friends were waiting, including Harold's wife Helen. Their faces revealed a bemused, and then shocked state-of-mind, because, just as Harold parked the truck, one of the tires went totally flat.

What would we have done if that had happened on I-80? How could we have unloaded the van? That brave tire paid the ultimate price for carrying our heavy equipment. I praised it for holding out so long. Then I opened a bottle of champagne. Of course, I felt the right thing to do was to buy four new tires for the truck. So I did.

Harold stayed several days and helped set up the new location. Before our 30 days had passed, our problem had been solved. We simply transferred our business into the revamped house. We didn't miss preparing even one meal.

The incident proved a blessing in disguise. Preparing for the move prompted a reassessment of our need for capacity. We were adding distributors in other towns. I felt we were on the verge of a growth spurt.

Our second office left us better situated. One reason—not to be taken lightly—is that I knew the owner—Kelly—would never kick us out.

When you're a young company, all that is required of an office is that it enables you to be productive and do your business.

We liked our location, though it later produced a serious problem. A fellow who lived with his sister across the street took exception to our presence.

The siblings in question had always lived in the same house, first with their mother, father, and an uncle; and now with each other, since their parents were deceased.

Sometimes we baked extra muffins, and gave some to the brother and sister, and other people working nearby.

The brother began to complain about the noise of our refrigerated trucks. I'm in great sympathy with people who like to live in the midst of quiet. But we were operating in a commercially zoned area, with a Buick garage across the street, and a Post Office to the south of our building.

Anyway, as time passed, the brother persistently complained, phoning me frequently, and standing outside to stare at our employees.

I got to thinking maybe we should move again. We discussed the possibility with many friends. As previously stated, Marseilles is a small town. Before long everyone knew what we were considering.

Most of the citizens did not want us to move. In fact, the townspeople presented us with a petition asking us to stay.

I didn't know what to do.

And then, all of a sudden, we were taken to court for the noise of our refrigeration. Three days of jury trial.

You know, it was a pain. But when your intent is pure, and your heart is true, good things always happen. People came out of the woodwork to help us.

The Post Office employees testified about the many frivolous complaints the brother had made about them. So did the proprietor and employees of the Buick garage. Other people vouched for us.

I liked the friendly support, but I wasn't sure what the jury was going to do. You never know. They might have wanted to award him something. I definitely disagreed. It wasn't the money. Goodness, we wouldn't have to personally pay. The insurance company had that responsibility.

So we could have settled without any financial pain, but that did not seem right. There was some pressure, but I wasn't tempted. The insurance company agreed with our position.

When all was said and done, the jury awarded him nothing. I was pleased. But the whole thing was hectic and stressful. I don't like wasting my time and resources on something irrelevant and marginal.

As I said earlier, the first phases of any project are strewn with landmines. It's almost as if a hopeful beginner has to pass through an initiation in order to escape the grip of petty, jealous, fearful, mediocre, negative, thinking.

We succeeded in freeing ourselves.

Yet I can't help but ask the common-sense question:

Why can't we all move forward together?

Chapter Twelve

Kathy Tuntland came on board in 1988, and has been vital to the success of our company ever since. Before she arrived, our growth had placed us in a challenging situation. Our continued success necessitated a continuing series of ever more difficult adjustments.

We were adhering to the highest standards in terms of menu selection, food preparation, and delivery. But a new degree of sophistication and professionalism on the business side seemed necessary.

I'm told that many entrepreneurs have trouble giving up real power in their companies. The idea is like a "baby" and they naturally feel they are the ones to raise their child.

Kelly and I taught our children to be self-reliant. We trusted them. And we had not been disappointed. At the right time, we had seen them leave the house, and make happy lives for themselves.

Maybe that's why I felt comfortable with Kathy. Or perhaps it's my innate understanding that leadership is part inspiration and part delegation.

I passed the test that faces an "idea person" when the time comes that she or he must surrender exclusive nurturing rights or be overwhelmed by the exponentially increasing administrative challenge.

I give most of the credit to Kathy. She's easy to trust.

Kathy has a degree in nutrition. She did her internship in school lunch programs. Until we started working together, I really didn't know that I needed someone like her as much as I did.

I know I'm getting ahead of myself here, but after learning my lesson with Kathy, I advise all our franchisees that the best kind of person to run their production is someone with a college degree in food science.

Kathy started when we were still in Marseilles, in Kelly's old office. Her chief responsibility was—and is—managing the nutrition aspect of our business. She oversees every aspect of our meal preparation, from menu selection to meal delivery.

During her first year, she and two other employees shared an office upstairs, directly above the ovens. Their work space was so hot their computer frequently overheated.

I don't think it was comfortable, but nothing deterred her. She didn't complain. She just kept working, making sure the meals were delivered healthy and fresh, and organizing our business in new and better ways.

One of Kathy's significant early contributions was to install an excellent labeling protocol. For some reason, the labeling "task" intimidated me. "How can we do that?" I lamented to Kathy. "We just can't!"

"Sure we can," she answered. And she figured it out, because she knew what was required. She also worked hard to increase her computer savvy.

Before long we were able to run improved ingredient analysis programs. Kathy was a big help early, and soon became an absolutely essential component.

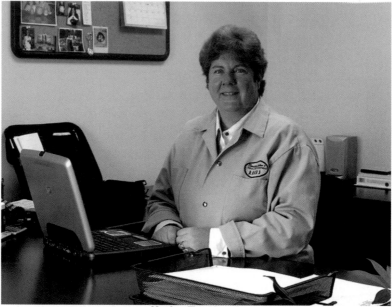

Kathy Tuntland

Meanwhile, more and more people began to purchase our meals. Advertising has a cumulative effect, and by now, we'd been on radio and TV for a while.

Orders were coming in from all over the Chicago metropolitan area, and we were in the midst of increasing our meal-making capacity, selecting distributors, and adding additional weeks to our menu rotation.

We have never in our history missed a meal delivery to a distributor. Our refrigerated trucks have completed every one of their twice-a-week scheduled rounds. Nothing stopped them. Not snow, not rain, not low carbs.

The biggest challenge came early on, when we only had one truck, and the extent of our determination might not have been established in the mind of our driver.

One bad weather morning he phoned me, and asked if he might delay his delivery until the snow stopped falling.

My answer, "Do you want me to drive?" Point made. He hit the road.

That is the last time any of our drivers—we now have sixteen routes—called to inquire about canceling (or postponing) a delivery.

Snow storms in Illinois are not daunting, in my opinion.

Of course, I grew up in North Dakota.

What I consider "bad road conditions" is when you have to drive fast to smash through the next snow bank on the highway. You must hit the bulked snow hard—like running through a wall.

In North Dakota, driving in snowy weather was like driving through a tunnel, because snowplows banked the roadsides with high white walls. When the wind blows during a snow storm, a driver can not see the road. Snow can come down so heavily that there are times people have to crawl out of their second story windows in order to leave their houses.

When snow falls in Illinois, I have been known to drive to Chicago to shop, only to discover that the clerks have not been able to come to work.

Our suppliers pride themselves on the reliability of their deliveries to us. One of them has only missed one day in the many years we have done business together. They pulled back because the Interstate conditions seemed impassable. But the sales rep who services us saved the situation. She loaded up her car and drove through the storm. Thanks, Julie.

Kelly and I put her up for the night, and the next day, as the snow continued to fall, our trucks were loaded and rolling.

Yes, their trucks pulled back, but ours made it through the storm.

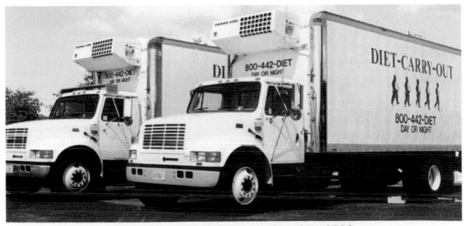

Diet-Carry-Out delivery trucks, circa 1990

Both our distributors and clients expressed their appreciation.

By now, Diet-Carry-Out had eight employees. One day I suggested it would be fun to go to lunch at the Ottawa Steakhouse wearing Groucho Marx disguises—you know, with the funny nose and big glasses.

We called the newspaper and told the assignment editor we were not going to eat our own meals for lunch. We were going to eat out, but in disguise.

Sure enough, a photographer showed up and took our picture. The paper ran it the next day, along with another story about how well the company was doing.

Nothing like a little fun and free publicity.

I believe it's absolutely essential that our company—any company for that matter—have a genuinely caring relationship with its workers. To me, the idea of grinding employee wages as low as possible is unfair, greedy, and gross.

There are no winners in a greed-driven workplace. Who can be happy and productive in such a vile environment? Nobody. Why would any good person purposely add unhappiness to the mix? Because of fear? Please. Grow some backbone. Do the right thing.

In 1987, we had a very good employee whose daughter developed some serious psychological problems and attempted suicide several times. The young girl had been darkly influenced by a wacky religious cult, and, though she no longer belonged, her thinking had been negatively affected.

Kelly referred her to several different psychiatrists. Before long she was heavily medicated. But she was not better. Nothing seemed to really help.

Beautiful girl. Not married. In her early 20s.

Her mother, one of our earliest employees, came to me in tears. What could she do to help her dearly beloved? She didn't know where to turn. Lately she'd been thinking it would be good for her daughter to get a job and spend time with people tuned into the workday world.

I wanted to help so I had a meeting with all my employees. "Look," I told them, "We know we can help people with the meals, and here's our chance to help someone by letting her come to work here. She's heavily sedated and may not be able to function like we might expect a new employee, but wouldn't it be wonderful if we could really help? Without your one hundred per cent cooperation, it can't be done. What do you think?"

Every single person at our company agreed: "Let's see what we can do."

The young woman came to work with us and stayed for years. It wasn't long before she no longer required medication. To the present day, she is doing very well. Presently, she makes a strong contribution to health care and our community by working as a nurse's aid.

Sure, it took extra effort from all of us to get her started and over the rough spots, but without a doubt—in the long run—she gave us much more than we gave her. Everyone—including me—gained an extra layer of satisfaction and happiness.

Try that in a greed-driven business.

One of the basic assumptions of our workplace has been to maximize trust. The same concept is found in every winning sports team.

I also don't think an employee should fret about the lifestyle or performance of any others. Diverting attention from the task in your hands is a sure-fire path to mediocrity…or worse. Focus!

In 1989, we moved again…this time to a bigger and better facility in Ottawa. Kathy Tuntland describes the period after this move as the "time we actually got organized and professional." If so, I think she was the main reason.

Good thing too. The business was continuing to grow, and so were our preparation and distribution challenges.

We had been delivering meals for four years by then. Wow! In a way, my voyage through these years reminds me of the railroad trip my fellow nurses-in-training and I made from Jamestown College to Cook County Hospital.

Our distributor ranks were growing. Many of them had customers who wanted us to deviate from our basic plan and follow some of the courses suggested by the marketing "experts" during our early days.

It's important to know what customers and distributors are thinking. We learn a lot from them. But it's essential to stick with a program in which you believe. If a suggestion—like providing menu options—was antithetical to our plan, and I knew we couldn't or wouldn't accept it, I made sure to let everyone know our reasons.

A person has to heed wisdom gained from experience, and a lot of mine had to do with being a mother.

And you know what? Running a company is really no different from raising healthy-minded children. You have to explain the "why" of your decisions.

For example, some of our distributors wanted to sell a five or ten meal weekly package. Sounds good, yes, but that's not our business.

We have to hold fast to our genuine mission.

The main reason I decided to start the company was to help people get results by improving their eating habits and helping them acquire a sense of proper portion size.

I knew it would take at least a week eating our food for people to make adjustments. That's why I designed the program to provide 21 meals each week—breakfasts, lunches, and dinners—and made it necessary for customers to order one week at a time.

If distributors just sold dinners, for example, the customer could undo the good of the evening meal by over-eating at breakfast and lunch. What is the possibility of good results then?

See what I mean? That's the "why" of our policy.

During the next two years our business flourished. Our customer base continued to grow, providing additional money for advertising. Which, in turn, fueled our further expansion.

Then, in 1991, the acquisitions frenzy that is such a troubling aspect of our economic system descended upon our doorstep. Campbell's Soup Company developed an interest in us.

The company's Head of New Developments brought many different people from Campbell's to Ottawa. Finally, I sat down to meet with them. Our attorney, Ed Sutkowski, of Peoria, was also present.

Ed had been the corporate attorney for the Marseilles Medical Clinic. Kelly and I had known him for years, and we trust both his advice and his ethics. Over the years, I have also received counsel from Mike Reagan, a local attorney who helps us with local matters.

I was reluctant to sell, my main reason for being in business, as I have already stated, was to help people eat healthy and get good results. Wouldn't a successful national company like Campbell's be able to fulfill my vision of a nationwide system of distribution?

Maybe. But we'll never know, because just as our negotiations were coming together, the president of Campbell's suddenly died. His death threw the company into some turmoil. I think a few development people may have been laid off.

Anyway, the deal didn't happen. I never learned the true reason.

One day the fellow who had been in the forefront of Campbell's negotiations with us—their former Head of New Developments—showed up in Ottawa. The fellow and his family—two wonderful little children—had moved here! I hadn't even decided to sell, and he and his wife were here to buy!

The short tale is that he eventually convinced me he could take our company national, and so I sold it to him in April of 1991.

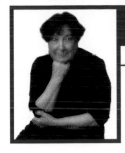

Isn't it sad many of us, including children and teenagers, see a sign proclaiming "Health Food Store," and believe that everything in that store is healthy?

People tend to believe that products are reliable merely because they are being sold. A more accurate sign might read: "Not Always Healthy Food Store."

Some hard-to-believe claims for benefits ranging from banishing cellulite to boosting brain power remind me of the purveyors of patent medicine and snake oil, two "supplements" of the 19th century.

But this is the 21st century, and perhaps our modern supplements can be of real value. I'm not from Missouri, but you still have to show me.

I would like to see the AMA work with the federal government to create accountability in the companies that are producing and selling herbal products and vitamins.

Testing needs to be a priority, since Americans spend more than $4 billion a year on supplements like ginseng, gingko, garlic, ginger, etc.

So far there is little scientific proof to support claims made by supplement manufacturers. This creates a danger that people will place trust in an untested remedy instead of seeking a doctor's help.

The FDA doesn't have the resources to adequately regulate supplements, and, incredibly, has the burden of proving a particular substance is unsafe, instead of making the manufacturer prove it is safe, which is how pharmaceuticals are handled.

There is no magic pill as good for you as healthy food.

Basically, the combination of unhealthy eating and reliance on supplements is, well, foolish.

(Continued)

A lot of people tell themselves: "I know I'm eating junk food. But I don't want to worry."

So they buy a bottle of multivitamins and think, if one is good, maybe three are better. Wrong! Too much can have a toxic effect.

Additionally, labeling is imprecise, and I have read of some frightening cases of people unknowingly taking as much as one thousand times the recommended safe upper limit of a vitamin or supplement.

Lax standards put consumers in an extremely dangerous situation, especially in the American sports culture where athletes and coaches try almost anything to gain a competitive advantage, even at the expense of their own safety.

Practically anyone can walk into a drug or health store and buy an unrestricted quantity of supplements, vitamins, and herbs. The government has been slow to regulate this industry, even though the health ramifications may turn out to ignite a national crisis.

Therefore, it is absolutely essential that we regulate ourselves. Parents, this especially means you.

My advice: Use your thinking rights.

Discuss vitamin pills or herbal supplements with your doctor before prescribing them for yourself.

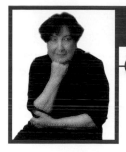

Use Your Thinking Rights!

PROMOTIONAL STUDIES & GENUINE FOOD SCIENCE

Too often the public is misled by so-called scientific medical studies.

One comes out supporting, for example, a particular drug that is being pushed by a manufacturer. Boom go the sales. All seems well.

Lo and behold, twenty years later a new study informs us that the original was incorrect. The use of estrogen to aid women during menopause is an example. The correction came too late for those who spent their money and trusted the drug.

We need to more closely examine the claims of "promotional" science. Consider, for the purposes of illustration, studies involving oatmeal. Does it really lower your cholesterol? Or is it the fact you are no longer eating bacon and eggs?

Many studies have been sponsored and designed with non-scientific goals in mind. I don't know how you describe such activities, but I think they are manipulative and shameless.

Seattle Sutton's Healthy Eating follows the principle of applying medical and scientific knowledge (as well as common sense) to the business of healthy meal preparation and delivery. We don't have any selfish reason to choose one food over another.

Therefore we crave reliable scientific information. Here's what we've learned. The best sources for trustworthy information are the American Dietetic Association, the American Diabetic Association, the American Cancer Society, and the American Heart Association.

Make sure that any science that influences you has the backing of one or more of these groups. Beware of many so-called "independent" studies. It's essential to know the sponsor.

Duke University, for example, conducted a well-publicized project which seemed to support the Atkins diet.

But I learned this research was sponsored by the Atkins Foundation.

Hmmm. Use your thinking rights.

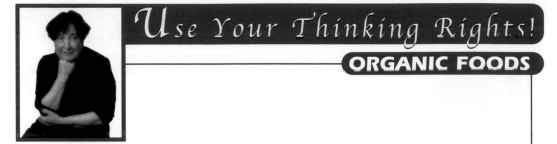

Here's a modern misconception: Organic food is healthier than non-organic food.

Why am I questioning organic superiority? Isn't organic food better for us because it is free of chemicals? Well, if it were, it would be. And that's a fact.

Many people believe that our fruits and vegetables should be grown without insecticides and other unnatural chemicals. They search the produce marketplace to find such products.

Unfortunately, a claim of organic doesn't necessarily guarantee an absence of pesticides, because chemicals can be transferred through manure.

That's the dark organic secret. If grown in manure, organic foods lose their "purity." Twenty-five percent of products labeled organic may contain pesticides.

Organic labeling criteria and certification began in 2002. Please be aware that the term "natural" is not regulated.

Products made with organic ingredients must contain at least 70% organic ingredients. Therefore, 30% does not have to be organic. This means that some—perhaps many—products that state they are "all natural" may not be.

What should we consumers do? Use our thinking rights!

As the Department of Agriculture points out, a label that says organic makes no claim that organically produced food is safer or more nutritious than conventionally produced food. No distinction can be made between organically and non-organically labeled products in terms of quality, appearance, or safety.

My husband told me that when he was young and hungry for an apple, he'd proceed cautiously because he worried about biting into a worm.

Today, if we bit into an apple and found a wriggler, we would be horrified that the grocer would stock such an item.

Worms no longer consider apples a safe haven. That's because of pesticides.

All in all, despite our good intentions, we may not be gaining much—except the possibility of worms—if we choose organic rather than non-organic.

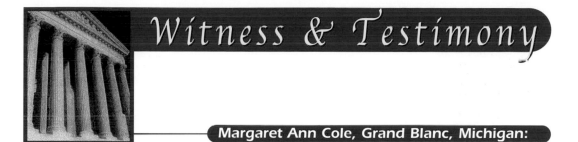

Witness & Testimony

Margaret Ann Cole, Grand Blanc, Michigan:

"My daughter had great success on Seattle Sutton's program. I thought it would be fun for the two of us to do this together. I have been on the plan for about four months and have lost 33 lbs! My cholesterol level has dropped from the 320s to 144. SSHE has truly given me hope when I just didn't think I had any."

Wynnette Cheek, Roswell, Georgia:

"I started the SSHE plan while visiting relatives in Chicago, and lost eight pounds in three weeks. Then I returned to Georgia, and learned there was no Seattle Sutton's there. I was heartbroken! But in January, 2004, I heard a radio ad for Seattle Sutton's of Georgia, immediately visited the website, found the distributor for my area, and ordered the meals. I'm now in my fifth week, and have lost 14 pounds. I am thankful for SSHE's meal planning and preparation."

Donna Gromek, Burnham, Illinois:

"My daughter Samantha is eight years old and was up to 135 pounds. I tried everything. Her self esteem was very low, and in school, kids can be cruel. I felt for my baby and wanted to help her. I heard a commercial for Seattle Sutton's. Samantha went on the 1,200 calorie diet plan and is averaging a weight loss of two to three pounds weekly. She is down to 117 pounds and her self esteem is through the roof. She loves the food and I love going to work knowing she is eating what she should be eating and not a fatty fried meal! I would recommend Seattle Sutton's Healthy Eating to any parent with a child that needs help on weight control.

Mary Anne Johnson, Champaign, Illinois:

"Seattle Sutton saved me!! I've been yo-yoing my entire adult life. Nothing worked long-term. Now I feel I can eat sensibly, have my hunger under control, stay healthy, and continue to do this the rest of my life. In just five short months, I've lost 68 pounds, 11 dress sizes, and gained self-confidence and health. I love the quality of the meals, as well as the freshness, and variety."

Witness & Testimony

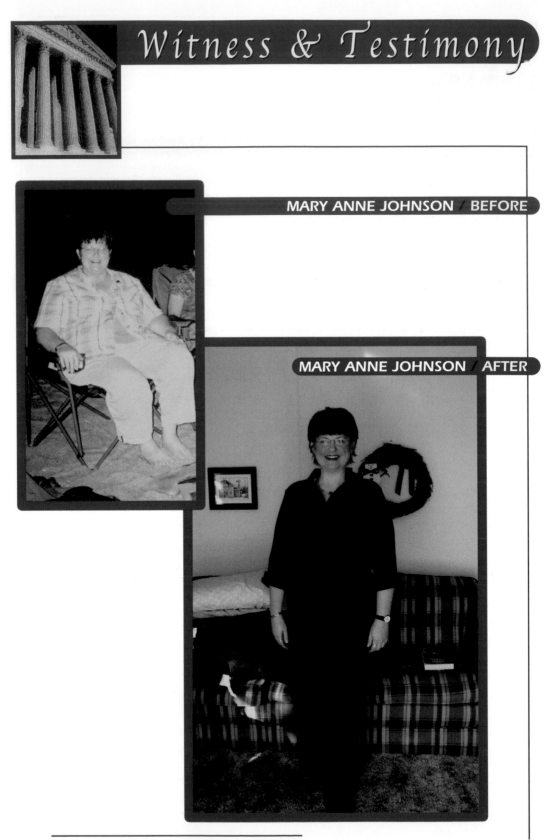

MARY ANNE JOHNSON / BEFORE

MARY ANNE JOHNSON / AFTER

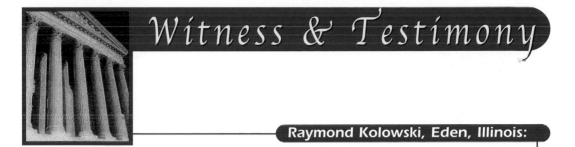

Witness & Testimony

Raymond Kolowski, Eden, Illinois:

"I started Seattle Sutton's program in April of 2003. I'm single, and it is so easy to go to the fridge and take out your meal. Heat it and eat it! And it's good for you. Previously, I did not eat my vegetables or greens. I would recommend Seattle Sutton's to anyone who values convenience and healthy eating."

Yvette Ramiriz, Omaha, Nebraska:

"I thoroughly enjoy the SSHE program. I have lost over 30 lbs and have tried new foods that I thought I didn't like or wouldn't enjoy. The opposite is true. I have too many favorites to list. It's easy to eat a Seattle Sutton's healthy lunch instead of a super size McDonalds, which had been my regular lunch routine."

Bette Resis, Chicago, Illinois:

"My doctor told me I needed to lose 30 lbs. I turned to Seattle Sutton. I never thought losing my first 15 lbs could make such a difference. My husband's friend was put on Seattle Sutton's program after a heart attack—so I knew it had to be healthy if a doctor recommended it!

Bob Henrikson, Highland, Indiana:

"When I began the Seattle Sutton's Healthy Eating program, I weighed 265 pounds and had Type II Diabetes. I was taking 1,500 mg of Glucophage daily to control my diabetes. After six months, I was experiencing low blood sugar, and within eight months was off all medication. My diabetes has been under control for almost a year. I have had a successful weight loss of over 50 pounds."

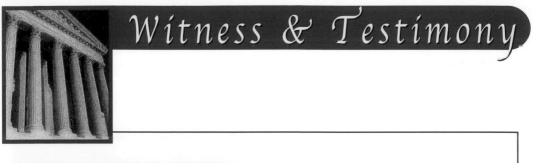

Witness & Testimony

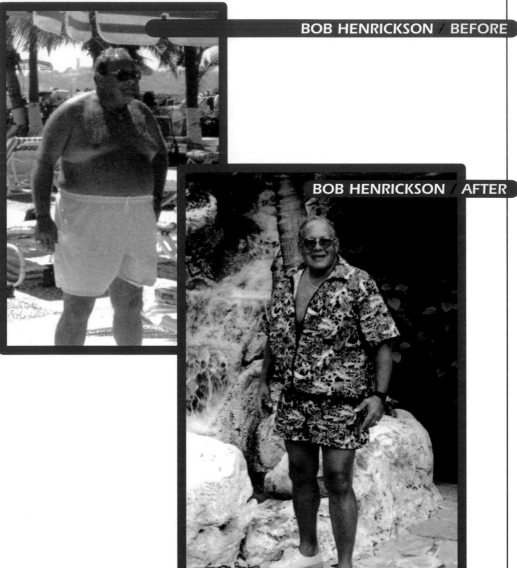

BOB HENRICKSON / BEFORE

BOB HENRICKSON / AFTER

Chapter Thirteen

Things went badly from the beginning. The new owner immediately embraced the marketing and distributor advice that I had disdained. And he allowed himself to be unduly influenced by bean counters.

Bean counting is a phrase that describes a process in which all the functions of a company are measured and interpreted by financial values. No other considerations are allowed. Statistics rule.

Evidently, the purpose is to minimize the "human" element. As if that's a good thing.

Well, the survey and statistics people may imagine that they can come up with all the right answers, but I don't agree. They certainly don't consider all the variables involved, because they can't. Even if they could, their criteria are financial, and, no matter what a bean counter believes, that doesn't feed the real bulldog.

Strange new company.

I remember being asked to attend a focus group. We hid in secret behind a mirror while people asked "a sample group" about the company's meals and food. The resulting report came to the exact opposite conclusions than what I had learned from my years talking to customers, distributors, and employees.

Believe me, I'm never going to do a focus group. You can count on it. Anyway, it seems sneaky to me—sitting behind a mirror so I can see them and they can't see me.

Of course, the survey statistics people think they are the smart ones, and anyone who doesn't pay them for their advice is "behind the times." If you have seen the movie, "It's A Wonderful Life," I'm sure you'll agree with me that yesterday's Mr. Potter is today's Mr. Bean Counter.

Heartless. Therefore, can't see the forest for the trees. Ultimately foolish.

Consider their impact on Diet-Carry-Out.

First the new owner changed the name of the company from Diet-Carry-Out to Freshly Yours. Okay. That's his privilege.

Then he altered our policy on food choices, and even included high-calorie foods like cheesecake and hot dogs that our customers need to avoid. Plus he offered a too-large family-sized portion.

Instead of having someone who knew the business answer the 800 lines, he used a phone bank service in Nebraska, with a staff of approximately one hundred.

Those operators, who may have been very good at their work, were only superficially trained—if that—in the business of Freshly Yours. They had no clue about our business. They certainly couldn't talk to our potential customers about our meals.

All they could do was keep a record: "This person called from this number, blah da blah da blah." Every day the answering service forwarded a record of calls.

By the time the company got around to following up these leads, it was already too late. Freshly Yours lost many potential customers because people contemplating a basic change in life don't like being treated in an impersonal manner.

During my days of answering 800 numbers, I routinely spent as many as 30 minutes talking with an individual caller, getting to know each of them, answering questions, developing a relationship. That contact was meaningful and helpful—exciting to the caller and me.

Under the new owner's system, a new typical response to an inquiry was: "We don't know anything about it, but give us your name, address, telephone number." Not very helpful. Frequently, potential customers were referred to the wrong "closest" location.

In addition to the changes listed above, chaos ruled the administration of Freshly Yours. The owner's office was a pit with papers scattered all over the floor. Worse, phone calls often were not returned.

A receptionist would place a note on the new owner's door, asking him to please call such-and-such distributor. He wouldn't.

Perhaps he was psychologically incapable because he thought the "boss shouldn't be bothered." Two weeks later the message would not have moved from its original sticker spot; a return call would not have been made.

Without a doubt, the new people radically altered the dream we had labored so hard and so long to bring into reality. It was a blow. On the counsel of Ed Sutkowski, I resigned from the board of directors.

The new owner never asked for my advice. Maybe that was on purpose. I certainly would have told him my thoughts in a direct and forthright manner.

The menu changes followed a predictable course all right. Only it wasn't the one prophesized by the surveys and focus groups.

Providing healthy meals no longer remained a priority. Basically, Freshly Yours morphed into a junk food catering service.

That change destroyed the business.

They should have used their thinking rights. By allowing customers to buy less than 21 meals a week, the company's ability to generate results disappeared. Customers who only ate dinners, for example, reverted to their previous eating habits for breakfast and lunch.

That is so obvious. To me, it is only common sense.

During my years at Diet-Carry-Out, I felt it was my responsibility to manage the company and keep it sound. When changes were suggested, I tried to think through the positives and negatives, and anticipate the consequences.

I expected the new owner to do the same.

Instead of eagerly accepting the opinions of a few vocal distributors and hired gun marketers, it was up to him to do a thorough analysis of each proposed new move before making a decision. He didn't.

If someone is managing many different details of a company, prior to any changes these questions should be asked: "Why didn't I do that in the beginning?" and "What will happen if I make a change?"

When I first started, I briefly imagined that every one of our procedures would be perfect, and we'd never have to make any changes. Of course, I quickly realized this assumption was a fantasy.

I'm willing to make changes if I'm convinced it's an improvement for our clients. A change might be difficult, but if it's the right thing to do, okay, go for it.

Sometimes people make changes for the wrong reasons, and I think that's what happened to Freshly Yours. The new owner didn't really want to be a healthy eating company, he just wanted to sell meals. Some high-priced marketing palookas and a few distributors convinced him they knew the way to increase sales.

Wrong!

Freshly Yours slowly slid down the drain. We watched its descent, knowing the end was near, although I don't know if its new owners had the same awareness.

Probably yes, because one day in 1992, as quick as they came to our little town, the family headed back East.

The fellow had the brass to ask me to manage the company for him. My attorney laughed with me at the offer. I wasn't interested in running his business his way. How would I know how to make decisions? By his values? Or mine?

I pondered the idea of taking over the company again and starting over. Can one jumpstart a derailed dream?

I still owned the headquarters building in Ottawa. One day, out of the blue, I received the news that a serious buyer had surfaced and had made a respectable bid for the property. If ever I had an opportunity to abandon my dedication to my idea, and resign myself to a life of rest and play, this was it.

My daughter Ruth had been a distributor for Diet-Carry-Out and Freshly Yours. She had watched the company self-destruct from her vantage point in Schererville, Indiana. Now she urged me to start over.

"Let's do this again, Mom. I'll help you however you want. You don't even have to pay me."

Quite a commitment. Inspiring. Thought-provoking.

I asked Kathy Tuntland to have lunch at our house. She had worked hard throughout the Freshly Yours debacle year. The shift in ownership philosophy had been difficult. But she had stuck it out, and done her best. Now what?

Kathy and I have never had any trouble communicating. I told her my plan. Would she like to join Ruth and me in rebuilding Diet-Carry-Out? If so, I'd like for her to buy stock and be one of the company's owners. Unfortunately, she wouldn't receive a salary for at least two years. Neither would Ruth nor I.

Kathy immediately said yes. How wonderful!

Working with Ed Sutkowski, I offered $50,000 for the equipment, all rights to the name Diet-Carry-Out, and the toll-free number 1-800-442-Diet (3438). I didn't want to buy their corporation, because it had incurred many liabilities, including borrowing quite a bit of money from banks.

At first, they resisted my offer. I think they were interested in bargaining, but it was hard to tell. They never attempted to convince me to meet their outstanding financial obligations. They did ask me to sell the company's assets piece by piece for them, but I wasn't about to do that.

Finally, a bank to which they owed money told them they "needed to accept Seattle's offer" in order to pay back their loans.

So they did.

After the purchase was complete, I received bills (to the attention of Freshly Yours) from advertising counselors—please!—out East, but it didn't take much to prove that the debts were not ours to pay.

Even though Freshly Yours left many businesses—our main providers included—with an unpaid balance, not one looked to me for payment. They welcomed us back with open arms. No supplier put us on cash-and-carry or anything similar.

Everyone noted that I—and the company while I owned it—had an unblemished credit record. We always paid our bills on time!

I restarted the business in 1993.

Selling—and buying back—the engine that incorporated my vision may seem sad, but in a very real way turned into a positive.

Sure, I made a mistake selling the company. Yet it's how someone handles a goof that tells the tale. Once again, I think parents are the shaping influence. How they react to their children's mishaps—how they help their offspring to succeed during a crisis time—is important. Lessons learned in youth are relied upon as guides during difficult periods in an adult's life.

As for our company, we learned for sure what "not" to do. We secured an absolutely clear understanding of what we wanted to do and what we didn't. We were strengthened in our belief that we were neither a caterer nor a carryout café.

Any lingering doubts about the value of "modern business applications" were removed. Our faith in our own judgment was reinforced.

Confidence was high!

First thing on our agenda was to give our building a thorough cleaning, and make any necessary renovations.

Second, we put our old policies and menus back in place.

Before long, we were organized again, and coming on strong.

In 1996, I changed the name of the company. Our franchise and patent attorney, Stuart Hershman, felt "Diet-Carry-Out" was too generic. He suggested we use my name. "It's unique," he said, "and we will have no trouble with the trademark." His comment reminded me of the cheerleader vote in Jamestown.

And that's how "Seattle Sutton's Healthy Eating" came into being.

Our "second time around" had the feel of starting over, but with the added advantage of knowing what we were doing.

We had faced the same challenges previously, and fought the same battles, and learned our lessons. We had a high level of confidence in each other, and in our business plan. We believed we knew what to do—and how to do it.

Using a sports analogy, it was as if we were an expansion baseball team that had been rookies the season previous, and still had won the pennant. Now, with a year's experience under our belt, we were going for our World Series rings.

Our business formula again showed its worth. Combining the power of advertising with the quality of our product launched us again into a winning cycle: more customers, more money for advertising, more customers, etc.

The next few years passed quickly. We had momentum. Many people now wanted to be distributors for us. Too many to accommodate. Early on we were just about begging people. But by the mid-90s, the situation had reversed.

Presently, Ruth has applications from about one thousand people wanting to be distributors. She allows distributors that follow procedures well to open a second location, and if that goes well, a third. A very few have been allowed to open a fourth, usually because they have family members to help them out.

Another of Ruth's responsibilities is training new distributors.

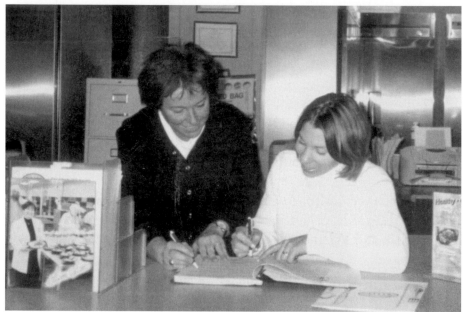

Ruth (left) is training Amy Moore, one of our distributors

At one such session, she showed her Sutton mettle. The new distributor had read the training manual, and seemed to know what he was doing. Good! Another zip code well covered.

At the appropriate time in the training, Ruth told the new recruit that he, like all distributors, would receive one order at a substantial discount.

We do that for all our distributors, because we want them to know our (their) product. It's never a problem. The majority of our distributors are former (and present) clients. They love the meals.

This fellow didn't agree. He said to Ruth, "I'm not into that stuff at all. I'm going to eat what I want to eat. I like McDonald's."

I am really proud of Ruth for packing up her materials and leaving. She told him, "This isn't for you. How can anyone sell our meals when they don't believe in healthy eating?"

He called me as soon as Ruth left, but I agreed with her assessment. We needed a distributor in his area, and he seemed like he would have been very good at sales. But neither Ruth nor I fretted about her decision.

It is the responsibility of the distributors to take orders from the clients and send them to our headquarters every Friday by noon, using either fax or email. Every order is a retail sale by the distributor, who is neither an employee nor a franchisee. They each operate independently, and pay us no fees for the right to become a distributor.

David Swartz, a gifted and valuable employee with many organizational and creative talents, tallies and processes all the orders so we know the correct quantity of groceries to purchase. Once we have that information, we get to work ordering supplies and preparing meals.

Distributors are almost always available by phone. That's good service and good business. We can't and won't tolerate distributors that don't meet their responsibilities.

Eventually, Kathy, Ruth, and I decided to ask Sarah to become part of the business. Our growth rate had increased the workload.

Sarah liked the idea, but, like Ruth before her, hesitated to give up her R.N. duties. Finally, inspired by the idea of working out of a home office and thus being closer to her children, she chose to join us.

I cautioned them that this meant that her husband, Bob, would have to be willing to accept many telephone interruptions on a daily basis. I stressed the fact that her purchase of shares and becoming part of company management would require weekend and holiday work.

Sarah and Bob discussed the possible pros and cons and, with Bob's wonderfully supportive attitude, the decision was finalized. I feel so fortunate to have two daughters involved, as well as my dear and trusted friend, Kathy Tuntland.

The rest of my family would probably be on board, but distance and other careers are important considerations. Peter's wife, Terri, can't wait to become a distributor once a franchise is sold in the San Jose or San Francisco area.

Chapter Fourteen

Many of our potential customers tell us, "Why didn't I call you a long time ago? Why didn't I know about you?" I don't think it's because they weren't paying attention. The average person has to hear about a new product about ten times before the message registers. That's why you can't get frustrated by running an ad and getting no response. Keep getting the word out, and everything falls into place.

Of course, the best advertising for us is word-of-mouth. A client does well, loses weight, feels good. Friends notice. Questions are asked. And we are the answer.

An advertiser like us must try many different types of media. It's important to ponder the circumstances in which your ad will be seen, heard, or read.

Everyone watches television, but quite a few people only listen to the radio in the car. Not everyone reads the newspaper, but some do.

Since different people are reached by different media, to figure out where to place advertising, you have to use your thinking rights. I think eventually you have to do a little of everything.

Begin with the simple and obvious. Most who are on our program are working people. That's why they are too busy to prepare their own healthy meals.

How can we reach potential customers in this demographic? I tell our distributors that everything works because we're getting our name out. But the main consideration has to be, "Will the person hearing the commercial be able to respond immediately?" That's right. The "instant call" is vital.

By that criteria, radio is excellent, because just about everyone has a cell phone. But what about movie theaters? The cost is low, but so is the chance for a viewer to respond. Do you think he or she will get up and go out into the lobby to call us?

No, they won't. So, except in a general branding sense, this is not a good option for our product.

Salesmen have tried to convince me to advertise on airport television. My response: "Well, when people are returning home, do you think they watch the terminal television? And if someone is preparing to leave on a flight, are they really interested?"

I don't think so. So that buy is not for us.

Some of our distributors have purchased advertising on the back of grocery store receipts, which I do not think is useful. Isn't it obvious? The people who have these receipts have just finished purchasing their food supply. Are they likely to call? No.

It's common sense.

I do believe in branding, but the method has to pass the "think test." Is it practical? Why will it help us?

Our top two branding successes are simple and effective. First, we use an easy to remember toll-free number. 800-442-Diet.

We had a choice. We could brand one number, or we could use a different one for each commercial. The latter would give us a tracking tool, but the former enables our advertising to have a cumulative effect.

We chose to brand our 800 number, and I'm glad. People don't necessarily have to look up our number. They've heard it many times.

As for tracking calls, I don't think it's worth the trouble. When we ask callers responding to ads where they heard of us, their answer now is usually something like "all over the place."

I still do not expend money or time for surveys. As long as the business grows at satisfactory average annual rate of 20%, and our distributors are on the right track, we know we're doing fine.

Distributors may call and report a good response from radio advertising, and ask for more. I hear them, and fully consider their requests, but there are so many variables. How much money, for example, has been spent recently on radio, as opposed to television and print?

The founder of a thriving enterprise must meet an essential obligation by anointing and training one or more successors. It's part of the healthy maturation of a business. As mentioned, I have heard anecdotes of leaders who had great difficulty surrendering their power. It's understandable, as I've mentioned previously. It's not been a problem for me, because I am good at delegating.

Recently, I have been training Sarah to handle our advertising.

This is the duty I've kept to myself the longest. Placing our ads is a big responsibility, because it energizes our business, and is absolutely essential.

I started with zero advertising knowledge and experience, and that proved to be my advantage because I didn't buy into a lot of the sales hype garbage. Sarah is also starting from scratch, though she has my experience to guide her. Like me, she was trained as a nurse, not a media buyer. It's a whole different universe.

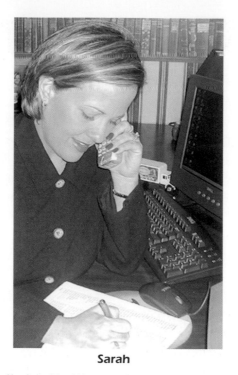
Sarah

Sarah can handle it. She'll soon be better than I am, and I'm satisfied with what my advertising purchases have accomplished.

When Sarah talked to her first television advertising salesperson, the sales gal tried a few tricks to get her to up our buy, even asking: "What's your total budget?" and "How much are you spending on station X?"

The right thing to do, of course, is to point out these are rude questions, and we are not obligated to respond.

Sarah did the right thing by refusing to answer, but when she called us to report the conversation, she expressed frustration.

"I don't know what to say," she said. "I'm certainly not going to give them the answers, but the inappropriateness leaves me speechless."

Kelly, listening on the other phone, had a suggestion: "Ask them what are they having for dinner, or their golf handicap, or how many pairs of underwear they own?"

Sarah laughed…and the lesson was learned.

They say that Abraham Lincoln used anecdotes and jokes to charm his foes and entertain his friends. It must be something in the Illinois water, because Kelly possesses the same talent.

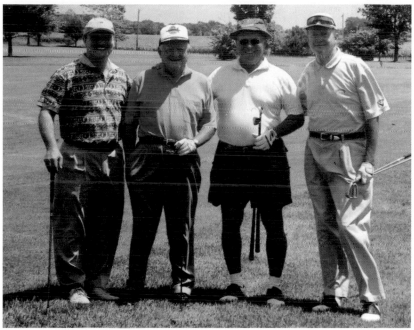
Community Hospital of Ottawa Golf Outing Winners
Drs. Giger, Sutton, Bettasso, and Lewis

When it comes to advertising, everyone has an opinion, and/or is trying to sell something which may or may not be valuable. One thing is certain: every aspect of advertising is important, because people pay attention.

For example, you may have heard the commercials I make with Ron Santo of the Chicago Cubs. A registered dietician came to me, and asked, "How can you be associated with Ron Santo when he is such a poor example of handling diabetes—drinking beer and eating hot dogs? Even when he gets serious and goes on Seattle Sutton's, he doesn't stick to it." I received an email making similar points, implying I shouldn't have anything to do with Ron.

Well, I don't agree. Ron is my friend and I'm on his side.

Everybody loves him, including the people at our company. Ron's a Type 1 diabetic who has lost two legs to the disease. He's a wonderful human being, and I'm sticking with him. Hang in there my friend!

Loyalty is important, and so is telling the truth.

I've continued to be part of our commercials because I still believe it's important that potential customers get a sense of a company's true personality.

A spokesperson is merely an actor delivering a scripted message. Thus, a commercial based on that approach is nothing but an act. If the act sells, fine. If it doesn't, the actor will be replaced, and a new script written.

Such an advertising message has nothing to do with the true value of the product, and, in my opinion, is designed to manipulate rather than provide reliable information. How can a consumer make an informed decision in such a circumstance?

As for Seattle Sutton's Healthy Eating, our approach is simple: present the facts of our program in an honest, straightforward manner.

Clearly, this is not universal.

In December of 2003, the Federal Trade Commission took a step to stop deceptive weight loss advertisements by issuing a "media reference guide." The guide describes seven phony diet gimmicks, and asks the media to be on guard against accepting such advertising.

We'll see.

Some people (and companies) will do anything for money, including publishing ads and promoting products which bilk and hurt people. Shame on them!

How much psychological, physical, and economic damage has been inflicted on desperate people who bought into fraudulent weight loss claims instead of relying on healthy eating?

Too much.

Sure, the deceived consumers could have used their thinking rights, but that doesn't justify fraud. As for Seattle Sutton's, we attempt not to advertise anywhere that promotes unreliable products.

FYI, here are the seven false advertising techniques flagged by the FTC:

Claims a product can cause weight loss of two or more pounds per week for a month or more without diet and exercise.

Claims a product can cause substantial weight loss no mater what or how much the consumer eats.

Claims a product can cause permanent weight loss (even when the consumer stops using the product).

Claims a product can block the absorption of fat or calories.

Claims a product can cause a consumer to lose more than three pounds per week for more than four weeks.

Claims a product can cause substantial weight loss for all users.

Claims a product can cause substantial weight loss by wearing it on the body or rubbing it into the skin.

Here are some copy excerpts from actual ads:

"Eat Your Way To A Trimmer You!"

"The Amazing Fat Sponge in a Pill."

"No Dieting. No Gyms. The Amazing Fattacker."

"Lose 30-40-50 Pounds. Works for Everyone. No Side Effects."

"A Pair of Earrings Could Help Me Lose 20 Pounds!"

"Take Pounds Off—and Keep 'em Off with the Singapore Slim Miracle Pill."

Aren't these ads preposterous?

Who could possibly be persuaded?

Anyone not using their thinking rights.

We can imagine the damage done. But, in my opinion, other "gimmick" diets also make misleading statements, even if their advertising doesn't make outrageous claims, and their intentions are good. Okay, now, what am I going to write next?

You are correct. The only way to lose weight is to burn more calories than you eat.

My husband, Kelly, tells me that some of his patients evidently still have a lot of willpower saved up—because they never use any.

Want to lose weight? Don't have enough willpower? How can this be true? Willpower is not inherited. It is a choice.

Use your thinking rights. Willpower is simply making up your mind.

Each of us—without exception—possess a will to live, so powerful that if we somehow actually truly lose it—almost impossible—we are likely to die. This will is strong enough to re-shape the way we eat, if that is our true desire.

The question is: How do we want to use this natural tool? To slog along? Or vivify our better dreams?

Sometimes a lack of self-esteem inhibits our use of willpower, and many of us can be strengthened by outside sources, such as a doctor or a mate. We may need to hear from a physician that, "You've got to lose weight to avoid a negative consequence," like having to take diabetic medication, or suffering congestive heart failure.

In the end, each of us has to individually find the inner resolve to do the right thing, and use our ever-present will to achieve our desired ends. There's no other way. This is both a benefit and a requirement of free choice.

The first dieting steps are the most difficult, because initial change requires the greatest effort. The temptation to revert to a previous habit demands (and expects) to be heeded. This is stinking thinking.

Overcome the initial psychological hurdles, begin to eat healthy and lose weight, and the path becomes easier.

Why? Because, by virtue of willpower, you have changed.

Habit is now your ally.

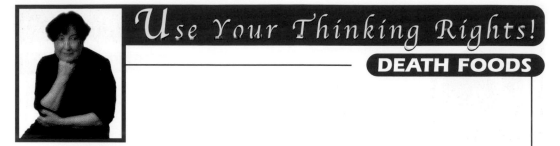

Are there certain dishes so unhealthy they deserve to be labeled as Death Foods?

Conceivably. Arsenic quiche, for instance. Lead paint pie.

But given what we actually eat, I don't know of any death foods. Not steak. Not eggs. Not doughnuts. Not even Twinkies.

With the exception of poisonous plants, there aren't any foods that need to be totally eliminated (at least that I am aware of at this time).

Moderation is the key. Once in awhile is okay. Use your thinking rights.

Perhaps you crave hash browns for breakfast. Hash browns have lots of calories and fat. So, if you are dedicated to healthy eating and weight control, you might be hesitant to eat one of your favorite foods.

I believe in most cases such a concern can become excessive. No need to banish hash browns from your life. Just limit the frequency, and the size of each helping.

A good balanced diet doesn't mean you have to eliminate your favorite foods. Healthy eating is a matter of portion, and preparation, and balance.

If we eat the same food for breakfast every day, that's not good. We require variety in our diets, and at the same time need to enjoy our meals.

Unnecessary sacrifice can produce a mind-set that says, "I can't wait for this diet to end so I can eat what I really want."

The key to healthy eating is simple. Meet your weight goals while eating the way you want to eat for the rest of your life.

How? Use your thinking rights.

Does it sound too difficult? Or impossible?

That's because you haven't begun.

I've seen it time and time again.

Once people start eating right, their previous unhealthy habits become an unpleasant memory.

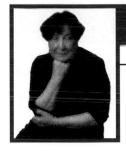

An analysis of the place of alcohol in a healthy diet also has to take into consideration some important non-diet elements. For some, drinking in moderation is difficult, if not impossible.

It is true that medical scientific studies show that a small amount of alcohol per day may be helpful in keeping arteries open. This seems to have something to do with decreasing the tendency of the blood's platelets to stick to the artery. Also, a little bit of alcohol dilates the blood vessels.

Other considerations—such as addiction—may of necessity prevent a person from any use of alcohol.

Any drinking, of course needs to be done in moderation. That's the key.

In my opinion, wine and beer are better alcohol choices. So called "hard" liquor is high in calories, and the calorie count increases because of the mixers used in cocktails.

Twelve ounces of beer, five ounces of wine, and one ounce of liquor (80 proof) all have about the same amount of alcohol, but the liquor appears to be absorbed more quickly and may put a bigger strain on your body.

Alcohol does add calories, and a first drink of the day sometimes encourages a second.

Always remember: portion control. Use your thinking rights before taking that additional drink.

Personally, I sometimes enjoy a glass of wine with my Seattle Sutton's Healthy Eating dinners, and do not feel that this conflicts with my dedication to healthy eating.

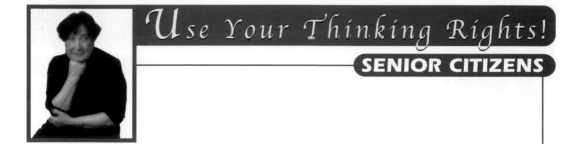

All of us are capable of using our thinking rights to better meet our nutritional needs, and none more so than our senior citizens.

Experience, after all, provides perspective, and is wisdom's mentor. Add to this axiom an understanding that the fact of survival to an advanced age is strong evidence of common sense and intelligence. Also, older people are already faced with the necessity to rethink and readjust their lifestyles.

Combine these considerations, and it's plain that senior citizens have a wonderful opportunity to eat healthier, and therefore increase the quality and quantity of their life.

Some people might have a misconception that people 70 years and older can't eat a balanced diet. Wrong. They should enjoy salads, fresh fruit, and a wide variety of healthy foods. Older people should not be restricted to just soft foods either. Fiber is important.

Many seniors focus too much attention on where they are going to eat. Dinner becomes the most important part of the day.

Well, I'm a senior citizen, and I like to eat.

I also like to work, and play, and think, and laugh, and walk. There's so much to enjoy, and healthy eating provides us the energy to live a balanced life.

The reason people gain weight when they get older is because they decrease their activity, but retain the same eating habits. They take in the same amount of calories, but expend less. What is the inevitable result? Weight gain.

This can be avoided.

Use your thinking rights, my fellow oldies but goodies.

If I may be allowed a short promotional tangent, I'd like to mention that many senior citizens, otherwise quite capable and self-reliant, find themselves forced to enter a nursing home because they are no longer able to shop for groceries and prepare meals.

Seattle Sutton's Healthy Eating to the rescue!

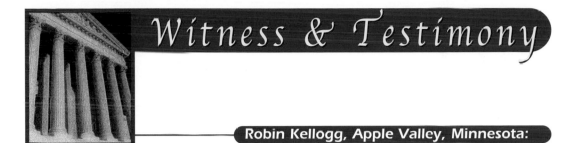

Robin Kellogg, Apple Valley, Minnesota:

"I am married with two children, and was not sure how Seattle Sutton's Healthy Eating was going to fit into my family life—but it has been so easy! Purchasing Seattle Sutton's meals is convenient and, all things considered, less expensive. Impulse buying is completely gone. I feel great and have lost 37 pounds...so far."

Lucinda M. Cordes, Davenport, Iowa:

"I have been a yoyo dieter since age eleven. I started dieting at 150 pounds and forty-three years later weighed 320 lbs. Then I discovered SSHE, and in seven months have lost 60 pounds. There is a tasty variety of gourmet food. I never leave the table hungry."

Larry & Rozanne Starkey, Bloomington, Illinois:

"We are so pleased with Seattle Sutton's Healthy Eating program!! Not only have we lost weight, but we have significantly lowered our cholesterol and triglyceride counts. Having the meals already planned and prepared is a wonderful convenience for a working couple."

Jill Jacob, Schaumburg, Illinois:

"When I started the program, I weighed 280 pounds. I lost 130 pounds in 13 months, and am not done yet. Already I can go into any clothing store and buy whatever I want. The meals are very good and the program is so convenient. I bring my breakfast and lunch to work. When I get home, I heat up my dinner, and that's it. I feel great and have a whole new attitude. Seattle Sutton's takes care of everything. It couldn't be easier."

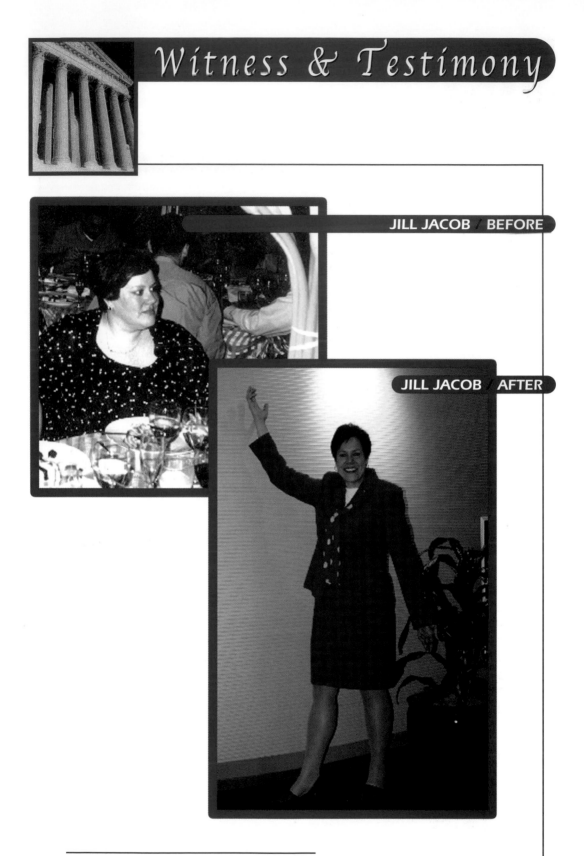

Witness & Testimony

JILL JACOB / BEFORE

JILL JACOB / AFTER

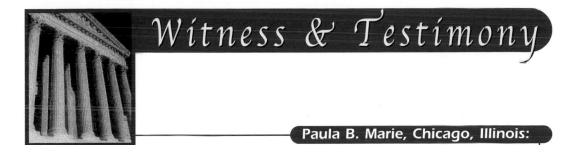

Witness & Testimony

Paula B. Marie, Chicago, Illinois:

"For more than twenty years, I have been a compulsive emotional overeater. When I came to SSHE, my weight had reached a high of 305 pounds. So far I have lost 40 pounds with Seattle Sutton's. This is the first time in my life that I have actually succeeded in losing weight, naturally and healthfully. Nothing has ever worked for me before. I am so grateful for this chance to create a new life for myself. I don't care about all the gimmicks out there—this works!"

Filomena Palermo, Oak Lawn, Illinois:

"I had been struggling with obesity for about 25 years. I tried everything—without success—until my children steered me to Seattle Sutton. I told myself it probably wouldn't work, but in less than a year I lost 122 pounds. I really enjoy the meals. It is not my Italian home cooked, but it is fresh, tasty, portioned correctly, and rewarding. I would recommend this to everyone who needs to lose weight or is going through health issues."

Patty Harris, Ottawa, Illinois:

"I have now lost over 50 pounds while on Seattle Sutton's Healthy Eating, with seemingly no sacrifice. I am amazed at how easily I lost. There are so many positive things about Seattle Sutton's Healthy Eating plan: convenience, ease of preparation, taste, and variety. I've tried to eat healthfully for years with little success. I think I felt the sacrifice wasn't worth it since I would always feel hungry and unsatisfied. Not with Seattle Sutton's Healthy Eating!"

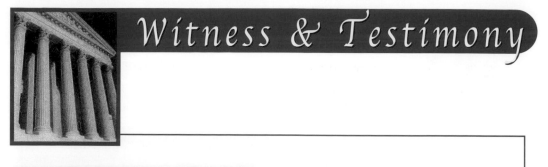

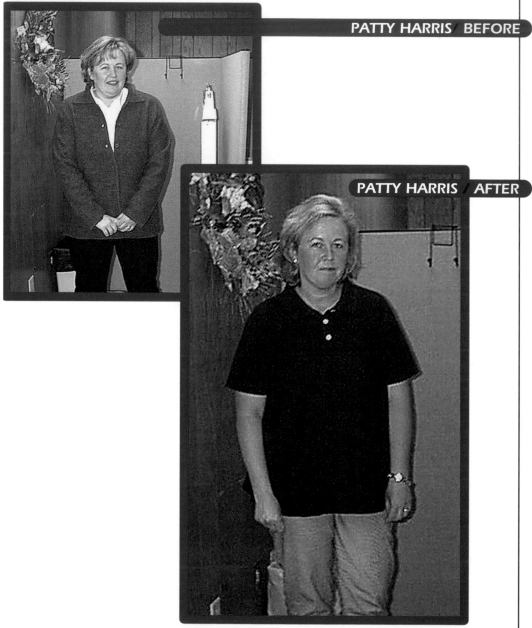

PATTY HARRIS / BEFORE

PATTY HARRIS / AFTER

Chapter Fifteen

When the company was smaller, I knew everyone involved, and we naturally became friends, and looked out for each other. Now, we have more than 130 employees, and are growing. Considering the food industry's high employee turnover rate and our continued expansion, maintaining that "one big family" feeling has become difficult.

That reality simply has to be accepted. Growth has both positive and negative consequences. That's how it is. Nothing can be done.

Something that remains in an owner's power, though, is to treat each employee with genuine respect. Goals can be established, and incentives offered, so everyone knows that if the company does well, they do well.

Most years, our employees receive a bonus if there has been company growth, all expenses have been paid, and productivity goals have been met. These goals have been reached every year.

I care about every employee, and wish I could know each individually. Though I am no longer responsible for the hiring, I am grateful for any time I am able to spend with them.

Christmas parties used to be held in my home. Our entire workforce and their spouses were invited. Year by year, more and more people attended, and our house was jammed with festive people.

Sarah organized everything. We all had a good time. I loved those gatherings. But our parties these days host about 200 people. Our house can't handle that many in winter. So that's a beauty gone. I truly miss it.

Don't get me wrong. We still have a company Yuletide gathering. We pick an attractive location, and let the good times roll. It's not the same, but it's still fun.

One year not too long ago, at our Christmas party, we hired a DJ, who presented a wide variety of music. Some of his tunes lent themselves to jitterbugging, and I had a great time dancing. Our employees are not shy about "tripping the light fantastic" with me.

One of them greatly admired my old car, a 1998 Lincoln Town Car. It was no longer new in 2002, but I still really liked it, and so, apparently, did he.

For months, every time our paths crossed at the company, he'd ask, "Seattle, how is that fine car running?"

At our Christmas party, I took the microphone and asked him to come up to the front. I noted that the company would be closed for two weeks during the holidays, and handed him the keys to my car.

"It has a full tank of gas. Go anywhere you want. You don't have to fill it up when you bring it back. It's parked right outside, in front of the main door. Have fun."

He walked out the door, got in the car, drove home to pick up his relatives, and continued to Atlanta for a visit with his Georgia family. When he returned the car after the holidays, he told me that all his relatives wanted to come to Ottawa and work for Seattle Sutton's Healthy Eating.

In 2002, we had our employee picnic at Buffalo Rock State Park near Ottawa. Unfortunately, it rained all day, but we had reserved a very large pavilion and had a dry picnic.

For weeks, I had been teasing Dale—one of our drivers—about the length of his hair. I assured him I knew how to barber, and asked for a chance to cut his hair.

Actually, it was only long in the back, and at work he tucked it under his hat. So it was no big deal, and I didn't really mind. But I enjoyed teasing him.

One day at work he came up and asked, "Seattle why don't you cut my hair at the picnic?" I agreed, and we decided to keep it a secret so we could put on a big show.

I took a hedge cutter with me to the picnic, plus a regular hair clipper, scissors, and several small ketchup packets.

I waited until the kid's games were finished and then announced, "Today we are going to do an extreme makeover on someone."

Wow, how the hands shot up. Everyone wanted to be chosen. But our plans were already made. I looked over at Dale and asked him to "come on up."

He sat down in the chair and I wrapped a half a roll of plastic around this neck, covering his entire body. People began to murmur. "What is going on?"

I picked up the hedge clipper as if to cut his hair, and pretended to accidentally snip his nose, at the same time discretely opening a ketchup package to simulate blood. The children laughed.

But I cautioned, "Do you think noses grow back?" I pretended to cut off his ear and opened a ketchup packet there.

By now the audience wasn't sure what to think.

"Let's go to the hair." I used the clippers to cut several inches, and held it up for all to see.

"Isn't this hair beautiful? You people might not realize this, but at my age, I am losing my hair." I tucked his hair under my hat, and cut another patch, and added it to my cache.

The audience seemed to be in a state of shock. They didn't know, of course, that Dale had approved this action. Soon enough, though, they noticed his wide smile and figured it out.

I ended up by giving Dale a crew cut, because, honestly, that's about the extent of my tonsorial acumen. Then I lathered his remaining hair with shampoo, and poured a pitcher of water over his head as a rinse.

"Oh my gosh, he didn't tell me he doesn't know how to swim."

Finally, to demonstrate my "Mod-ness," I colored his hair pink.

The audience roared, and applauded wildly when I announced that Dale and his wife had earned a trip to anywhere in the United States.

Why do something like this?

First, he asked me.

Second, I like to soften the divide between ownership and employees. This is only truly useful when both groups hold the interest of each other, and the company, in their hearts.

Employees expect more money when they do a good job. Excellent! I agree. The key to being a good employee in our environment is to do better than expected. You will be appreciated and moved forward.

As any good business owner knows, no matter how fair and reasonable the management approach, some employees will try to take advantage. A recent study revealed that 17% of employees don't even try to do good work.

Our approach reduces that percentage, but does not eliminate it. We try to help our employees understand that someone cheating us is also cheating them.

Yes, some of our people don't do so well in their work with us, and a few don't give a fair effort. We react accordingly. The good ones, however, are promoted, rewarded financially, complemented frequently, and supported fully.

My head driver was married with two beautiful children. Unfortunately, problems developed within the marriage, and divorce seemed the only answer. He was heartbroken.

One day he called me while driving his route. He was very upset. I felt so bad for him, and at the same time grateful for his trust. At his request, I called his wife, whom I knew well, and tried my best to help them work out their marriage problems.

But reconciliation seemed out of the question, so he filed for divorce. I met with his attorney, and even helped with some financing. When his case went to trial, I made sure to be present in the courthouse. He received residential custody of the children, and that's good, for he is an excellent father.

For the sake of the children, he and his ex-wife remained in touch, and this is fortunate, because now they have a good relationship. When he is making his deliveries the children stay with her.

I'm glad I was able to help. You have to go beyond the basics for a loyal employee who does all the right things for the company.

The same is true for a loyal manager and owner.

Kathy Tuntland: "When I started working for Seattle in February of 1988, I was pregnant with our daughter Shelley, who was born in May.

"Almost immediately, Seattle provided me a computer for my house and gave me every opportunity to work at home. Back in 1988, that was kind of unusual, so she was a trendsetter. I'm grateful for her style, because I've been able to raise three children, and do my job here."

Thanks Kathy, but I don't think there's anything special about what happened. It's only common sense. Family is first. Then, now, and always.

Many working mothers have a hard time not feeling guilty. I guess it's natural. I felt it when I worked at the medical clinic.

Kathy told me, "When I'm at the office, I feel like I should be at home. When I'm home, I feel like I should be at the office. I'm dedicated to both wholeheartedly."

It's a woman's dilemma, and each of us has to work it through as best as possible. Exercise your thinking rights!

I'm never one to give much power to guilt, though. What a waste!

I can't praise Kathy Tuntland enough. Year after year, she meets her responsibilities, and more. Often she is in the office during Christmas break, maybe even on Christmas day, organizing everything so we can resume cooking in an orderly manner, and doing what needs doing. I even caught her mopping the floors to avoid a delay in moving into our new facility.

Oh my gosh, it makes me feel bad to think about her missing family time. Wait a minute! Do I sense guilt?

Yes, I do, and maybe it is not a complete waste. On Christmas break, 2003, I sent Kathy and 20 members of her family to Hawaii. She deserved it. And, whew, I feel better. So long, guilt, goodbye.

Kathy is excellent at delegation. Her trusted and invaluable assistant is Tammy Blacklaw. Tammy is intelligent and talented. Kathy has often remarked to me about the tremendous work that Tammy does. She's a real help to all of us. And that's the truth!

Delegation of authority is recognition of limitation. Being that we're all human, and therefore limited, proper delegation is wisdom in action.

With no food or business background, I knew I had to surround myself with people like Kathy, conscientious about doing things right, and well-organized.

I value organization, and that's reflected in every aspect of our company. When our employees come to work on a specific day, they know exactly what their job is going to be. Our five-week menu rotation allows for exact planning. Every fifth Monday is exactly the same, and every fifth Tuesday, and so forth.

Kathy understood the importance of organizing the company, and its working schedule. She worked hard to bring the company in compliance with federal standards.

We're USDA licensed. Our facility, our trucks, our labeling, and our distributors are in compliance. Our trucks can cross state lines, which means we can take better advantage of our capacity.

Can you believe we have a USDA inspector based in our facility? We built a very nice working space for her. She uses it as her regional headquarters, while working with us and other companies in our area. But her office is on our premises, and we're proud of providing that service.

It's all part of doing the right thing. A reputation we've earned.

Gosh, we don't have to advertise for employees. Most of our applicants are referred by a current employee. We ask, "Is she (or he) honest? Do you want her (or him) working beside you?"

The usual answer is, "I've known her for 20 years. Her family lives down the street from us."

That's the advantage of operating in a small town. They know us, and we know them.

Not everything is roses, of course. Or even radishes.

When a problem arises with a customer or employee, our first response is to address it immediately, and let everyone involved know what we are doing.

We listen to all sides, and make our perspective known. Usually that's enough to solve the problem and show the complainants that they have a voice that's heard.

Sometimes it's not enough.

When we receive a call from a disgruntled client, we take it seriously. We listen carefully, and we evaluate about what we're hearing.

I do not easily tolerate a complaint I consider to be dishonest. That's why Ruth handles this part of the business.

She immediately phones the servicing distributor, and repeats what we have heard. "This person called. This is your client. This is what was said."

If the story told by the customer is more believable than the story told by the distributor, then the latter must apologize and fix the problem. If not, a change will be made.

Many times the distributor does provide another—and often more credible—explanation. That's when we have to make a hard decision about whether or not to dismiss the client.

That's right. Sometimes the customer is wrong. When this happens, the best way to protect the company is to end the relationship.

You see, not having contracts benefits everyone, including Seattle Sutton's.

My distaste for "participation contracts" is personal. I wouldn't sign one myself, and knew this at the moment of the project's inception, and made it part of the deal. Despite pressure to the contrary, we haven't changed.

I have negative feelings about contracts required by other companies selling gimmick weight loss programs.

First, they don't work, and are harmful. Second, the dieter comes to realize this. Third, an extended contract is not fair, and adds an unfair psychological and financial burden.

Some companies are afraid to operate without contracts. They want to eliminate the risk that people will try them for a week, and then leave.

We don't operate in fear our customers won't be satisfied. No contracts. Order the meals a week in advance. Eat them or not. Reorder or not.

We do have an advantage. Most people, once they have tried us for a week, never forget us.

Some of our customers buy our meals as a gift for someone who has just been discharged from the hospital.

Or someone nursing a baby.

Or elderly people who are home bound and find it difficult to shop.

For example, one of our distributors, Toni Smith, of Lansing, Illinois, reported that she sold twenty gift certificates in one day.

To be totally accurate, though, I need to mention that some of our distributors have come up with a proposal that is somewhat similar to a contract.

A distributor may know someone who is determined to stay on the program for many weeks to come, perhaps to lose 50 or 100 pounds, or because of an enjoyment of healthy eating.

In that case, because we know a customer has made a free choice to be on the meals, the distributor can offer a discount for multiple week pre-payment. We at headquarters permit such a transaction. It's a financial benefit for the client.

Some might argue that this is like a contract, and at some obscure level, perhaps it is. However, I believe it is substantially different because it is only available to someone who has already made a personal commitment to continue.

A free will agreement is not the same as a an obligatory contract.

Someone asked me: "Is Seattle Sutton's Healthy Eating, in any way, involved with pyramid marketing?"

The answer is no. No! Unequivocally no!

Chapter Sixteen

My belief in the value of delegation increased in November of 1999, when I was diagnosed with breast cancer and had a modified radical mastectomy. It's not something to be taken lightly, but I was highly confident it would amount to nothing more than a bump in the road.

I've been on tamoxifen, and also had several doses of chemotherapy. The chemo made me feel rotten! Really bad! So I queried my oncologist about its value. In my case, I asked, how much may chemotherapy help prevent further spread? His answer? About 2%. Not enough!

Too much pain for too little gain.

No more chemo for me. I'm glad I made that choice because I have had no further problems. I really don't worry about it. I think having the surgery was the right thing to do, although it greatly concerned my family.

My three daughters camped out in the hospital, and made me feel so happy it couldn't help but have a positive impact on my health. It didn't take much time for me to jump back into my normal routine.

Paula told me, "I don't know of anyone your age that ever recuperated so quickly from this surgery." Her sincerity comforted me.

Like I said, a bump in the road.

Several first cousins and my sister died of breast cancer. I knew my mother would be very concerned when she found out about my situation. So I didn't tell her. I think I worried more about that than the cancer.

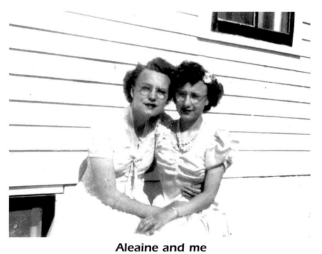

Aleaine and me

Of course, Mom did find out and asked me about it. I re-assured her that science and medicine had made major advances in breast cancer therapy since Aleaine's death. She was glad for me, but sad, again, for my sister.

The episode did remind me that the company I built had to be able to carry on without me. That's when I started delegating the phone system—and other duties—to Ruth and Sarah.

I miss that 3 a.m. ringing phone sometimes, but I know the callers are in good hands.

Prior to the next annual distributor meeting, I had to make a major decision. I like to recap the previous year at these meetings, and let our people know about our plans for the upcoming annum. These gatherings are always upbeat, exciting, and inspiring.

Likely, rumors of my illness had passed through the distributor ranks. I wondered if speaking to them about my surgery would be the right thing to do. Finally, I decided to tell them that I had been diagnosed with breast cancer, had surgery, and was fine.

It went well. Candor drains the poison from the sting of rumor. The distributors appreciated knowing the facts of the situation. Telling the truth is a wise choice.

Ruth has continued her careful selection and expansion of distributor locations. We now have approximately 200 in place, including those in Illinois, Wisconsin, Minnesota, Michigan, Georgia, Nebraska, Indiana, and Iowa.

Each distributor is an independent businessperson. They buy the food from us (or the franchise holder in their area) at a discount, and sell it to their customers.

Our distributors make no product investment because we deliver the first set of meals with an invoice, which they pay when we bring them the week's second set of meals.

While the company has the major advertising responsibilities, distributors also run their own local ads.

There is some turnover in our ranks, because that is human nature. My philosophy: If someone doesn't want to be a distributor for us, I don't want them.

Customers who become distributors because of a positive reaction to the company and its meals tend to be happy in their work, and bond well with us.

The vast majority of our distributors fit in comfortably with the company's program and philosophy. People of good will—who do the right thing even in difficult circumstances—have an affinity for each other. I like the fact that my company provides them with a way to make a living and please their conscience.

I don't allow our distributors to act as counselors, because they are not registered dieticians. If any of our clients feels a need for counseling, we recommend they see a doctor or a registered dietician.

Many of our distributors are nurses, and likely they could give useful advice. But the fact still remains: they are not professional dieticians. So the counseling ban applies. Simply put: we don't want to take a chance that one of our people might give a client erroneous information (about weight loss, for example).

The reason for this policy is not complex. We have several fields of expertise: menu analysis and selection, food preparation, delivery, and distribution. We take satisfaction from knowing that the people who order our meals are actually learning to eat right and control calories.

Not included in the list of our strengths is counseling. Since we're not trained, we should not do it. Therefore, we don't.

We gained additional credibility in the professional community because we don't allow our distributors to be counselors or sell nutritional supplements.

As hard as it was to make our independent sales force understand the value of those policies, they certainly worked out well. We receive many referrals from doctors, nurses, hospital discharge personnel, and dieticians.

We have to continually resist the idea of support groups. Some of our distributors pressure us. Our answer is always no. Without knowledgeable guidance, support groups are like internet chat rooms—an unending source of false information.

If you decide to attend counseling sessions of any sort, be certain the counselors are truly qualified. Make sure of their training and credentials.

When it comes to nutritional guidance, doctors or registered dieticians are my recommendation.

I also admire support systems provided by companies like Weight Watchers, who absolutely know what they are doing. I have often wondered if we could combine our food with their counseling.

No disrespect, because Weight Watchers does many things well, but providing freshly prepared meals is not one of their strength areas. Just like support group discussion is not one of ours.

I know that much of what I'm writing may seem like bragging. Probably it is, even though I don't intend it that way. I admit I'm proud, so please accept my apology for being prideful.

I am anxious to describe us as we are now, since you already know how we began. We're still on a path to an unknown destination, but we've reached a new level. Perhaps my description will inspire and motivate, if nothing else.

Being aligned with so many wonderful people is one of the most pleasant aspects of the continued unfolding of Seattle Sutton's. Here are a few examples (I easily could list dozens):

One of our distributors, Gail Caplinger, runs three offices, two in Illinois (Rockford and Roscoe), and one in Madison, Wisconsin. Working with her husband, Mark, she finds special meaning in her work.

"I love hearing the success stories," Gail said. "One young man, who lost 94 pounds, told me he felt like a new person. I have also seen diabetics find success in controlling their sugar levels."

I might blush to repeat her next comment, except it is not about me. It reflects the company.

Gail told her local newspaper: "Everyone associated with the company is very nice and helpful."

Another distributor, Eileen Spevak, a registered nurse who operates in the Illinois communities of Plainfield, Oswego, and Aurora, credits the success of her business to the consistent quality of the meals, and her belief in the program.

"I need no sales experience to sell something I can personally endorse," Ms. Spevak said. "I have seen first-hand how my own clients improve their health. Diabetics control their blood sugars, individuals decrease their high cholesterol levels, and many lower their blood pressure."

By eating our meals, Eileen herself lost 67 pounds in eight months, and decided to become a distributor. Since then, still on our program, she has not regained a single pound.

Jim Witczak, of suburban Chicago, is a very successful distributor with several locations, including the Oak Lawn, Burbank and Bolingbrook areas. He sent this note to Ruth:

"I just wanted to thank you for all of the opportunities you have given me, and I want you to know that I will never let you down. I am having so much fun selling meals and growing the business. We are helping so many people with their health and losing weight. I feel really good about what we are doing."

Another distributor of note is Sherry Garrett, who has an office in Moline, Illinois, and another in Bettendorf, Iowa. "There's no need for grocery shopping or counting calories," Sherry told the local newspaper. "We do all the work for you."

Sherry understands.

By organizing and applying our resources (in harmony with our fundamental principles of healthy eating) to the challenge of preparing more than 150,000 meals a week (and rising), we are able to plan, shop, cook, package, and deliver fresh, healthy meals to our customers.

Our distributors furnish their own office, coolers, phone system, and delivery vehicle. They order from us by noon every Friday, so we know how many groceries to buy, and meals to prepare during the next week. We order, cook, bake, package, and deliver accordingly.

Fifty weeks a year, without fail, twice a week, our refrigerated trucks take to the highways. When our drivers arrive at the various distributor offices, it is usually late at night or early in the morning.

Though the distributors are almost never there, the drivers have a key to every office on their route, and are able to take the meals inside and store them safely in coolers.

The temperature in the truck must be correct…and so must the temperature in the coolers. Every step is carefully controlled.

We are extremely careful about food safety, and are constantly monitoring conditions in our kitchens, during our packaging, on the trucks, and in the coolers. That's why our meals stay fresh.

If something is amiss in an office, the driver does not hesitate to call the relevant distributor. When a cooling problem is discovered, an immediate solution must be found! In fact, I encourage contingency cooling plans.

Clients receive 21 meals a week, nine on Monday and 12 on Thursday. They don't have a free day to eat "whatever they want" and undo the good we do for them.

Distributors are in their offices from 3 p.m. to 7 p.m. on Mondays and Thursdays. That's when our clients pick up the meals. Of course, our distributors are available by phone seven days a week.

If any prefer not to be accessible by phone, they should consider another line of work. We always stress, "Have your cell phones turned on. It's important. For example, what if a client's delivery time needs to be changed?"

Our people must meet the needs of our customers. After all, isn't that one of our foundation principles? Yes!

New distributors, seeking new customers, sometimes disagree with one or more of our policies. Once they have been in business for some time and are serving a larger customer base, they begin to appreciate the utility of our design.

Sooner or later, they experience an "Aha!" moment, and realize our consistency is our strength. If food choices and fewer meals were permissible, a distributor wouldn't be able to serve a large customer base for the same price.

We'd have to charge three times what we charge now. That's sky high, and not our style. We've had only one price increase in the last 13 years.

Besides, I've witnessed the disastrous consequences of those policies. Never again!

I have resisted every overture to place our meals in grocery stores. I don't want that. Can a store clerk have the same relationship with our clients that our distributor does? The answer is obvious.

Recently a distributor told me that one of his clients (in Wisconsin) felt so overwhelmed with her problems that when she picked up her meals, she stayed an extra hour just to talk.

Our guy listened. The conversation had nothing to do with the meals. She needed someone to hear her story. No big deal. No high drama. No life or death. One person listening attentively and compassionately to another in a time of need. Salt of the earth. I love it.

Here's another "feel good" example: One of our distributors recently reported that an obese woman, upon learning of Seattle Sutton's Healthy Eating program, cancelled her impending stomach-stapling surgery.

It costs a little extra to have the food delivered to your home by a distributor, but many people like the convenience. Others like to drop by the distributor offices. Many hang around to chat.

Frequently, real friendships are formed. Once a distributor called me to report that one of his customers had survived a difficult experience, in large part because of our company.

This distributor was delivering meals twice a week to an elderly customer. A relative had assumed the financial responsibility.

Attempting to make a delivery and receiving no answer, the distributor became concerned and called the supporting relative. Sure enough, the customer had fallen and was near death. Summoned by our good fellow, help arrived, and tragedy was averted.

Not all our interactions are so dramatic, but they still demonstrate the personal side of what we do. For instance, one of our distributors delivered our meals to a woman with Parkinson's disease. She felt so comfortable with him that she requested his assistance with her earrings.

Coordinating advertising reach with "covered" distributor territory is a difficult challenge. It's wasteful to advertise in an area that the company can't cover. Yet many of our advertising buys cannot be focused on just one area.

Placing ads with Chicago Tribune, for example, or WGN radio and TV, gives us a wider "reach." Advertising with these media is always very effective.

We assign our distributors by zip code. That's how we advance– one zip at a time. Potential customers "appear" in uncovered zips. So distributors "stretch" their territories for a while, driving long distances to deliver to a few customers. As the customer base expands, someone in the new territory inquires about becoming a distributor.

We take our time and do all we can to make sure we place the right people in the right areas, and that proper headquarters management and product procedures are in place to service them.

We know what we're doing, and we're on friendly terms with our consciences, fortified by our ethical hygiene.

We've advanced beyond the power of the bean counter world, but occasionally still take cannon fire across our bow.

As a result of one such volley, Seattle Sutton's Healthy Eating no longer trusts or relies on Dunn & Bradstreet. I have been told this may be a growing trend. Perhaps it's for the best. Their rating system can be ridiculous.

Here's an example:

We make a fair profit every year, which we use to upgrade our facilities, equipment, trucks, etc. We aren't required to do this, but we think it is better for our company and our customers.

We also bonus employees, management, and ownership. By the end of December, we typically don't have an overly large amount of money in the bank. This is fine, since we are an "S" corporation.

Our company always pays its bills on or ahead of schedule. Every bill, every month, every year. We pay promptly for our advertising, equipment, trucks, groceries, etc. There's never been a time we couldn't afford what we needed. The company has no loans, no debt, and no intention of acquiring any.

A dream come true? We think so.

In 2003, after a ten-year stretch in which we never failed to pay our bills on time, and our revenues expanded approximately 20% annually, D & B gave us a "Poor" composite credit rating.

Who are these people? Have they misjudged any other companies?

Enron comes to mind. I did some investigating. Several months before their collapse, D & B gave Enron a score of 78. A Dunn & Bradstreet employee told me that eighty is excellent. Seventy-eight is the very high side of "Good." So much for Dunn & Bradstreet's "information."

Though their approach irritates me sufficiently to reference in these pages, I know that D & B has little, if any, effect on our company. We don't need to borrow money. We're not looking to be acquired. Everyone with whom we do business knows and supports us.

But the picture of our business, which they have the audacity to show the world, is completely inaccurate. To make it worse, they gave me the runaround when I called to try to set the record straight.

D & B puts me in mind of the kinds of companies that promote gimmick diets. Promises, promises, and more promises. Broken by performance.

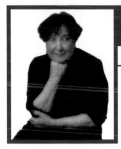

Some school soda dispensers are being replaced with vending machines dispensing healthy foods like fruits, fresh carrots, and juices.

It's a good start. Kids should be drinking water or healthy juices. But why stop with getting rid of soda? While we're on the topic, let us consider the whole idea of school lunches.

Where did the belief originate overvaluing the nutritional importance of a hot meal? Whether we eat something cold or something hot, all food is the same temperature during digestion.

Our school boards, with good intention, have made the idea of "hot lunches" more important than the real goal: feeding children healthy food.

Let's not kid ourselves. School lunch programs are embarrassing nutritional failures and do not provide our children healthy, well-balanced meals.

The current system also is wasteful and, therefore, not a good financial bargain. Hot lunches cost way too much, and that's without factoring in the long-term health care expense generated by the treatment of diseases caused by obesity.

Here is an idea to improve the eating habits of our student population, and, at the same time, free up much-needed educational funds.

Why serve hot meal choices that many children won't eat?
Be smart. Use your thinking rights.
Eliminate hot lunches.
They are unnecessary!
And, as presently distributed, too often unhealthy!

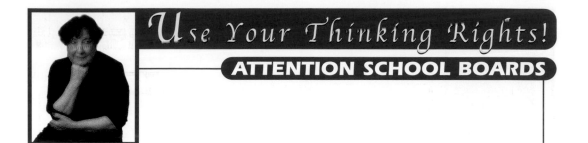

How much better if students were offered a peanut butter, cheese, or cold turkey sandwich every day, with fresh fruit, juice, or milk? I think we can utilize our knowledge of nutritional science to plan a healthy "cold" lunch regime.

Furthermore, let's take out ALL vending machines; eliminate ALL other options. That's the ticket to healthy eating.

I repeat. No more hot lunches! No more vending machines with sodas and junk foods.

Attention school boards:

We can save billions of dollars, and use that money to improve our educational system.

Better pay for teachers. More teachers. More educational resources.

Prevent the elimination of sports, and band, and other after school activities!

Board members! What are you waiting for?

Students can make their own sandwiches, and the school can provide the supplies. If necessary, one of the first things children can be taught in kindergarten is how to make their own sandwich, including what kind of bread to use (whole wheat).

Teachers, too, need to set an example. I read that a school board removed junk food vending machines from all the system's buildings, and some teachers brought in boxes of doughnuts on the first day of school.

Please!

Did they think the kids weren't watching?

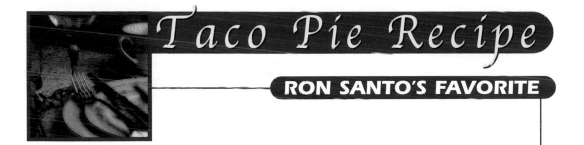

I can't write a diet book without including at least one recipe.
So here's Ron Santo's favorite, our Taco Pie.

Acapulco Taco Pie Recipe

Yield: 15 Servings

2 1/2 Pounds Ground Turkey
3/4 Cup Chopped White Onions
2 1/2 Tablespoons Chili Powder
1 Cup Green Chili Peppers
1 3/4 Cups Skim Milk
1 Cup + 2 Tablespoons Bisquick
3/4 Cup Egg Substitute
1 Cup Diced Tomatoes
6 1/4 Ounces Shredded Monterey Jack Cheese

Brown ground turkey and onions.
Drain.
Stir in chili powder and green chili peppers.
Place the meat mixture in a sprayed casserole pan.

Beat skim milk, Bisquick, and egg substitute until smooth.
Pour into the casserole pan directly over the meat mixture.

Mix together diced tomatoes and cheese.
Add to casserole pan.

Bake at 350 degrees Fahrenheit until a knife comes out clean.

Cut, serve with salsa and chips and enjoy!

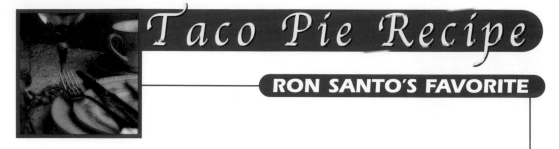

Taco Pie Recipe

RON SANTO'S FAVORITE

ACAPULCO TACO PIE

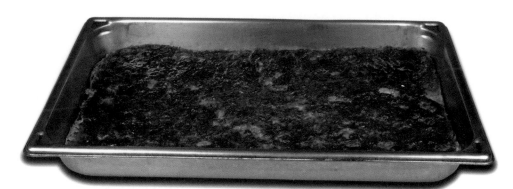

IN OUR KITCHEN

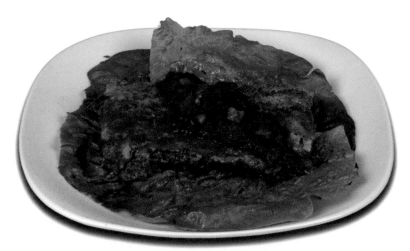

ON YOUR PLATE

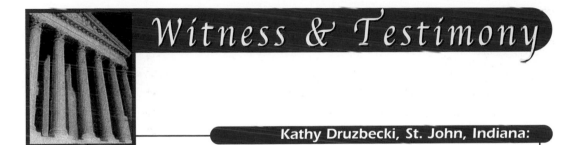

Witness & Testimony

Kathy Druzbecki, St. John, Indiana:

"I began just over a year ago and have lost 50 lbs. Several people at work who were originally quite skeptical are now interested in the program. The thing I like best is that I am not a cook, and with my work and a family, have very little time to put together a healthy weight loss program. With SSHE, all the work and planning has been done...and the weight just melts off."

Laura Hoffman, Moline, Illinois:

"I have had a weight problem since my late twenties. My dream was to win the lottery so I could hire a personal chef to make me healthy great tasting low-fat meals. Well, we all know the odds against that, but I found a way! I lost 52 pounds my first year on Seattle Sutton's Healthy Eating. It is the easiest plan I have ever followed. In addition to the weight loss, I have reduced my cholesterol to a normal level, no longer have stomach problems, and my backache and sore knees are in the past."

Susan Braun, Bolingbrook, Illinois:

"I've lost more than one hundred and ten pounds on the Healthy Eating program. It's been easy to follow, and I've never skipped a meal. Its been fun changing from a size 26 to a size 8, and buying new clothes along the way. I like the compliments from people who knew me when. It's been a life changing experience."

Witness & Testimony

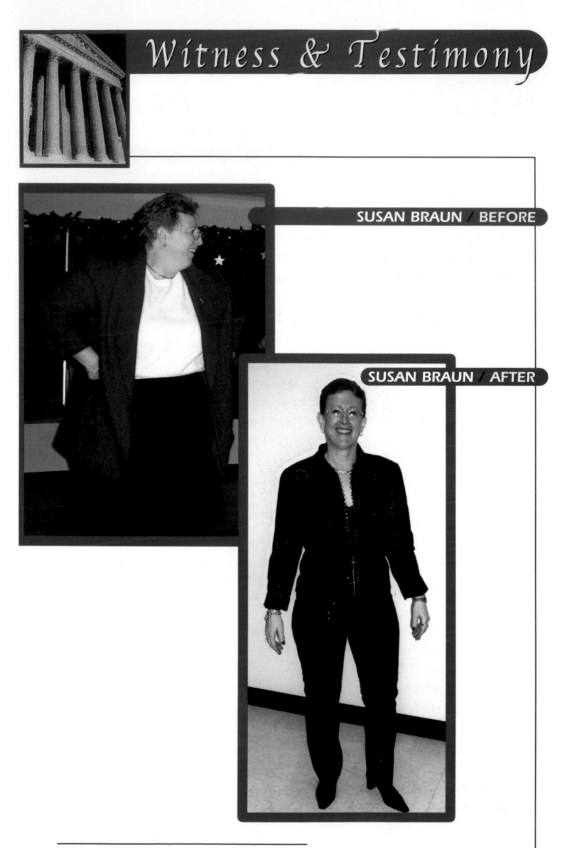

SUSAN BRAUN / BEFORE

SUSAN BRAUN / AFTER

The Seattle Sutton Solution

Are you finding it difficult to eat healthy, enjoy your meals, and lose weight? Seattle Sutton's Healthy Eating has a time-tested solution. No gimmicks. No tricks. No fad diets. No yo-yo.

Our program handles every step of the meal preparation process the right way, using scientific research, common sense, and a genuine respect for the needs of our customers. The Seattle Sutton solution is trustworthy because of its unmatched reliance on medical and nutritional science.

Here's how Seattle Sutton's Healthy Eating works:

We design, research, taste-test, nutritionally analyze, prepare, and deliver 21 meals a week to each of our clients. We have developed a five-week menu rotation, so meals are only repeated ten times a year. Our clients supply their own skim milk.

Our meals are fresh, delicious, and healthy. We do the planning and shopping, always using quality food and healthy ingredients. Friday is the day we take orders for the next week's meals, prepared in our own kitchens.

We bake. We cook. We package. We deliver.

Each client has an option to participate in our 1,200 calories-per-day plan, or our 2,000 calories-per-day plan. Portion size is the difference.

Our refrigerated trucks deliver to our distributors twice a week. Every distributor has a cooler system to keep our meals fresh. Our clients can pick up the meals at the distributor's location, or arrange to have their meals delivered.

Quality and freshness control are closely maintained during every step of the process. Seattle Sutton's Healthy Eating is dedicated to delivering healthy, fresh, and tasty meals.

All our clients need do is take the fresh meals from the package, warm in the microwave as necessary, and serve on a plate (whenever possible). Many breakfasts ad lunches don't need heating.

For further information, call 1-800-442-DIET (3438). Or visit the web site: www.seattlesutton.com

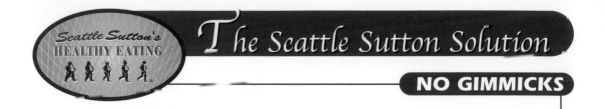
Seattle Sutton's Healthy Eating
Annual Growth By Client Count

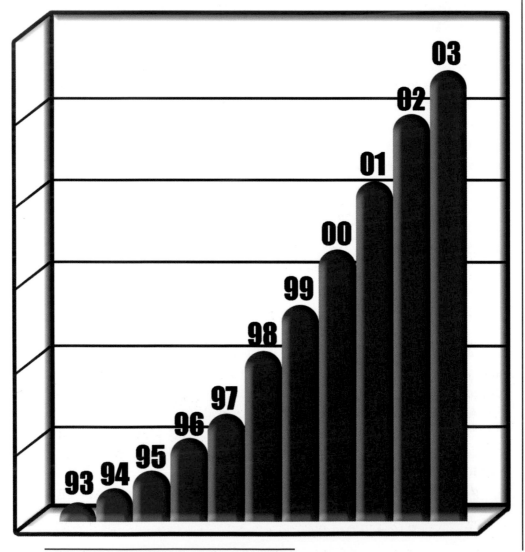

Chapter Seventeen

People anxious to lose weight frantically grasp at anything new. A lot of people have told me, "I have tried every diet."

Their desperation is an extra incentive for us to do our job correctly. We are fortified by the knowledge that our plan works in the short and long term.

We began in 1985 with a 9-day menu rotation cycle, and slowly expanded to 35 days. Each meal is repeated 10 times a year. We never deviate from our principle of keeping our meals sodium restricted, low in cholesterol and fat, and calorie controlled.

When we decided to go to a 35-day cycle, the process took time. Every Friday Sarah came to our headquarters with prospective meals she'd prepared in her kitchen. She brought breakfasts, lunches, and dinners, all of which satisfied the company's healthy eating criteria.

Which left the taste test.

We—some employees included—sampled her offerings, and noted what we liked best. Sometimes we'd say, "This might work if a few changes were made." Some meals were vetoed immediately. "I don't like how that looks," someone might say. "Neither do I," agreed another.

After reaching consensus on the worth of a meal, we stored it in a refrigerator for a few days. We placed it in a delivery truck. We evaluated how it microwaved. After each step, we held another taste test.

If the results were satisfactory, then Kathy Tuntland and Laura Farjood (our registered dietician consultant) went to work on portioning and further analysis.

Our meals are designed to meet the basic nutritional needs of any person, regardless of age, sex, weight, or general state of health. Simply put, we serve people what they should eat.

I retain an intense interest in the progress of food science, read test literature and professional magazines, and have an ongoing dialogue with various experts, dieticians, people in our company, and, of course, Kelly.

My objective is to be alert for anything science is learning about food. When something new is revealed, I use my thinking rights to try to get a handle on what it really means.

After this new information is evaluated, and if it is found relevant, we do our best to apply it in a practical way.

To give an example of our process, when we expanded to five

weeks, we decided to include a "Polish pierogies" meal, with a turkey sausage on the side, plus sauerkraut, and horseradish sauce.

At first, we tested pierogies—pastas stuffed with mashed potatoes—from a larger supplier, but they had far more sodium than we allow. It seems to me the bigger the food producer, the more junk in the ingredients.

We did some arduous detective work, and discovered a very small company that made them to our requirements. Naturally, we felt like Lieutenant Columbo at the conclusion of a successful investigation.

But the mystery was not totally solved. We spent weeks trying to find a low fat, sodium-restricted turkey sausage that fit our guidelines. None appeared to be available.

Finally we decided to start from scratch. We approached a nearby turkey farm and laid out our requirements. They listened to our need, and found a way to meet it. Now they make delicious turkey sausage that satisfies our specifications. No junk!

We were unsuccessful in finding a sodium-restricted sauerkraut. Even brands that described themselves as such were not low enough for us. So my husband and I tried an experiment.

We boiled chopped cabbage, added a little vinegar, and, eureka, very low sodium sauerkraut. That formula is now our staple.

When we began in1985, we made most of our own food, even our own crackers and mayonnaise. It is hard to overstate the difficulty in that era of finding companies preparing healthy food.

Like vistas perceived through the window of a fast-moving train, the situation has changed.

Presently, though we still cook and bake most of our food, we have arrangements with smaller providers for specialty items, and buy the vast majority of our ingredients from one of two huge suppliers.

Either could meet our needs, but we prefer the competitive aspect as a natural way to regulate prices, and double our protection in case of emergencies. It's no exaggeration to say we enjoy working with both companies. They are part of our research team when it comes to finding exact needed ingredients.

When we make a menu change, and decide to outsource the preparation, we ask one (or both) of our main suppliers to find a provider.

Typically, they search until a possibility emerges, and then approach the prospective vendor with this message: "If you produce a tasty, high-quality, healthy eating product, you will have an ongoing order from Seattle Sutton's."

Our suppliers help us enforce our specifications. Our rules, for example, ban artificial sweeteners. No food dyes. No MSG. Basically, no harmful additives.

Unfortunately, we can't get around using some hydrogenated fat. It's in so many foods that it can't be totally avoided. We are careful to keep the percentage very low. That's why we bake many items on our menu from scratch.

Industrially prepared pastries, bread products, muffins, and the like, use hydrogenated soybean oil as an ingredient because it is less expensive.

Hydrogenated fat is definitely a hazard. I don't know why companies are willing to risk the health of their customers just to increase profits.

Because we have a regular menu rotation, our food needs are predictable. A supplier purchases what we require in bulk quantities, and stores them in a large warehouse.

If we were to buy individually from each of our many vendors, we'd have nonstop deliveries at our back door. We might go crazy!

Before we put something new on the menu, our suppliers make certain it is available to us in Illinois, and to our franchises, currently in Minnesota, Michigan, Georgia, and Indiana. This is essential because our franchises must replicate our meal schedule exactly.

We also use both major suppliers as a front line of quality control. They sample the ingredients, and if something is amiss, often catch the problem and make the adjustment. Sometimes a provider will start out at one quality level, but over time the quality erodes. We expect our suppliers to stay alert.

Of course, we know we're the final line of defense, and are constantly testing and analyzing. It's comforting, though, to know we have allies.

One of our main concerns is portion size, more difficult to achieve in practice than in theory. Take the fresh baked sweet potato, for example, which used to come to us in different sizes.

An accurate count is easy, but portion consistency can be a real problem. Also, sweet potatoes tend to shrivel in the baking process, especially the smaller ones.

Our customers are no dummies. If two people in a family are on our meals, and one gets a bigger sweet potato than the other, well, does that sit right? If our portions are sized differently, our clients could logically reason, is our calorie count reliable?

Here's how we solved the problem.

One of our suppliers found a company that produces a round and thick center cut sweet potato. We bake and cover their cuts with an orange glaze. It's a better fresh baked sweet potato, for sure, and consistently portioned.

The quality of our food improves, our calorie count is reliable, our problem is solved.

I don't think we're going to add any more weeks to our menu rotation. Our customers eat the same meal only ten times a year now. Think of an average unhealthy eater's fast food repetition cycle. Fifty times per year? One hundred? Two hundred?

Instead of adding another week, we're going to concentrate on making every meal as perfect as possible. There will always be menu improvements. Our company will never be stagnant. We constantly monitor nutritional research so we can keep improving our program.

All our improvements must pass a taste test, survive Kathy's computer analysis and portioning allotment, and be okayed by our registered dietician consultant.

If approved, a new item faces a final test. Kathy describes it:

"We have to be able to prepare it in quantity without using too much intricate hand labor per portion. It has to fit into our production schedule. Do we have enough oven space and pans? What about kettle room? Sometimes we juggle meals from week to week to fit our schedule and resources."

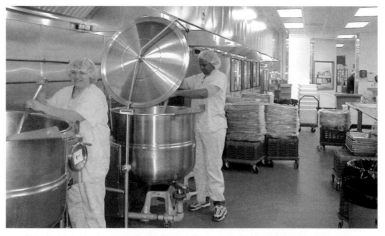

**Tina Neumann and Queen Carver prepare vegetables in
two of our 60-gallon steam kettles**

Besides the food analysis and preparation schedule, labels have to be changed, the packaging manual updated, and the ordering procedures kept on track. It's difficult for others to understand what it takes to implement any change, even a minor one. Thank goodness Kathy is exceptionally capable.

After every change, Kathy's assistant, Tammy Blacklaw, notifies our franchisees so that their kitchens can keep pace. A lot of back and forth ensues, but it is essential. Of course, our guiding principle is healthy eating. And we believe in providing food variety, and a well-balanced diet.

Right now many people are boarding the "no carbs" diet gimmick train. Let me state unequivocally: I believe this is unhealthy eating, and a fad diet.

I despise fad diets, which I define as any form of eating which cannot be maintained over a lifetime.

I think that some of our customers become bored if they eat our meals from the package. Presentation is definitely an important aspect of food enjoyment. My suggestion to our distributors is to ask their clients to please remove a meal from its packaging, put it on a nice dinner plate, and heat it up.

That's what I call gourmet.

Some of our meals, like our turkey parmesan with asparagus and roasted potatoes, have not changed since we began. My favorite is the orange-glazed Cornish hen with wild rice, baby beets, and cranberry relish. By the way, this is the only meal we serve that includes a bone. Many of our clients have expressed their fondness for this dinner.

Our spaghetti is delicious. We prepare it with a tomato meat sauce, a celery cheese casserole, and a poached cinnamon peach. That's a really good meal. I also like our fish almandine dinner.

One of my preferred lunches is BBQ on Texas crust served with fresh carrots and grapes.

Truth be told, I like every one of our meals. It's nice to anticipate a tasty delight coming up on the menu, though.

When someone says to me, "I don't know if I'd like this because I'm a fussy eater," my response is, "Great, if you're a fussy eater who likes good food, you'll enjoy our meals."

We exclude pork and red meat to take advantage of the greater ease of measuring fat and cholesterol in poultry.

We serve things like French crepe, pizza, stuffed shells, and meat loaf, so it is in no way accurate to think of our program as a deprivation diet.

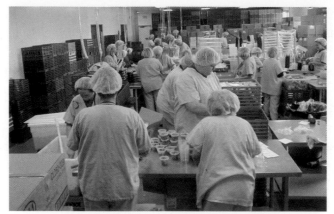
Here's where we package our meals

One of our clients has been on our meals for more than 300 weeks. She reports that she never tires of our food, and anticipates staying with the program for as long as she lives.

We surprised her with a bag of Seattle Sutton's caps, pens, note pads, water bottles, a wristwatch, and a wall clock. I like taking the extra step. People appreciate the unexpected bonus.

Some people ask, "Why do I have to eat your meals seven days a week, three times a day?" Well, the answer is one word. You've heard it before.

Results! I'll make it twice as easy to understand. Results! Results!

Measurable success is as important to the customer who wants to lose ten pounds as it is to the one who wants to lose one hundred.

Our customers have tremendous results, if they stay with the program for longer than a week. Some people do try for a week, and then discontinue, saying, "It's not for me."

Okay. That's fair. Don't like our healthy meals? So be it.

Usually, though, our customers stay with us at least five weeks, and the results are wonderful. Some go off for awhile, and then return.

Everyone can lose weight and feel better—men, women, all different age groups and body types.

We've had some clients who shed as many as 13 pounds in their first week. But that is because they had been eating high sodium and had edema. When they started on our program, they had significant fluid loss, which accounted for their weight drop, but, in truth, only signaled that they were now ready to lose real pounds.

Many of our beginning female clients order the 1,200 calorie a day regime, and stay on it until they reach a weight loss goal. Then they switch to the 2,000 calorie plan. If they go a little wild on a vacation and gain a few pounds. Then they use the 1,200 to get back to normal.

Whether it's the Type 2 diabetic lowering blood sugar, or an obese person losing pounds, or someone seeking weight maintenance, our program delivers results.

We have had much success with many Type 2 diabetics, because weight loss (in almost all cases) is the only thing that will help them if they are obese.

But a Type 1 brittle diabetic has to carefully correlate their insulin dose with their carbohydrate intake. Many times a registered dietician will inform Kathy that a more complete (instead of average per day) analysis is needed. Of course, we supply that information upon request.

I also know we have helped a lot of people who might be placed in nursing homes if it weren't for our program. Because we take care of their planning, shopping, cooking and delivery, we lift a very heavy burden from their elderly shoulders. We have helped a lot of people stay in their home.

Controlling calories is the problem. Ask yourself: "Did I stick to 1,200 calories today, or did I eat 3,000?" The latter number is usually the honest answer.

It's hard, it's difficult, it's frustrating.

Let's face it. If you are baking your own muffins, and smelling them in the oven, how many will you eat? One? Or six? Gulping down the latter number is more likely, even if it takes you a couple of days to get there. Too many calories.

Without good results, people become frustrated, and are not able to sustain their good intentions or their diet.

Many of our customers like to dine out once in awhile. That's okay. We provide some guidelines, which, if followed, keep the program on track.

For example, if dining out means you end up with an extra one of our meals, why not treat a friend? Or freeze it for later.

When you're in the restaurant, don't let all the options keep you from eating healthy. You can order lower calorie items, like breast of chicken and baked potato. Broiled meat of any kind is a good choice. And fish, of course. Remember the importance of portion size, and be moderate with things like butter and sour cream.

Another advantage of our no-contract approach:

If a client has something special on the calendar—perhaps a

cruise—they can skip a week or two and then re-order the meals when they return.

Our advice:

Hold your weight while you're off having fun. Resume your weight loss when you get back home.

We close for Christmas and New Year's. No food deliveries for two weeks. Our employees have a paid vacation. Other than that, it's a straight and steady flow. Ten five-week menu rotations per year.

When we first initiated this annual two-week break, we received many calls from elderly people informing us how much they depended on the meals.

We put on our thinking caps and tested which of our dinners best withstood freezing. Now, prior to our last delivery of the year, a customer can order ten extra dinners to freeze, a basket of fruit and juices, and our homemade sliced bread, and cream cheese.

My husband and I order this extra meal package to help carry us through the holidays. I have some meals in the refrigerator right now, so if you're hungry, come on over. Call first! (This offer is only valid for the first ten readers to apply.) Hah!

By the way, after more than 18 years of being on our meals program, I had my yearly physical in December of 2003. Not only is my heart in excellent shape, my HDL is 54 (normal is between 35-60), my cholesterol is 174 (normal is between 120-200), my glucose is 85 (normal is 70-110), and my triglyceride is 93 (normal is 30-200).

What's interesting about these numbers is that I'm the same age—72—that Dr. Atkins was when he died. I guess it's fair to say we each followed our respective diets.

Whenever one of our customers loses more than one hundred pounds, the local distributor informs me, and I call to personally offer congratulations. Then I send a check for $100 with a note of praise.

If someone were to tell me that she followed our 1,200 calorie a day program for a week and didn't lose weight, my response would be, "You are either cheating or sleeping all day."

Fact: If someone eats 1,200 calories a day, and gets out of bed in the morning and carries on a normal routine, that person can't help but shed pounds. Additional weight will be lost if the day includes a walk of twenty minutes or so.

The more calories are expended, the more weight is lost. There, I wrote it again! Not only does it feel good to reiterate, but writing burns calories. So does reading.

Once I made a presentation at a convention of several hundred registered dieticians. They allowed me to show my meals and speak for a few minutes.

A renowned obesity physician specialist made the keynote speech, and afterward, accepted questions from the audience. One of the dieticians asked about a patient who kept a list of everything she ate, and, according to her records, ate a maximum of 900 calories a day.

Yet she hadn't lost any weight!

The dietician asked the doctor if he would accept the woman as a patient. He paused before saying, "I can't help her."

In other words, he knew that the woman in question was not being honest. Probably she ate when she was hungry, but failed to record many of her calories

That's the cheating game losers play.

And I don't mean losers of weight.

Chapter Eighteen

Throughout this book, I have been candid about our business procedures. Some of my friends have suggested it would be better if I weren't quite so open about how our company operates...because this might give a potential competitor valuable information.

I hear that argument, and realize it has merit. But we are strong now, and I don't fear competition. Why should I worry? We're way ahead of everyone.

Anyway, the idea is to make healthy eating an easy option for as many people as possible. Would it be so bad if other companies helped us meet this goal?

Once in a while I read about someone in California or somewhere trying to develop a healthy food delivery business. So far, such efforts have based their strategy on advice from bean counters—the same approach that doomed Freshly Yours.

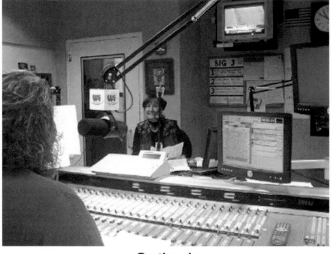

On the air

By telling it "like it is," I hope to be helpful to other good people who are considering bringing their own ideas into the world, and who share our goal of helping people.

Our basic mission has never changed:

Improve people's eating habits for life.

We arrived at our present prosperity and prominence by being open, and not surrendering to fear, so why should we change?

Because we have something to lose? I'm a conservative person, but I don't value negative thinking.

This is America, and if you have a dream, pursue it. It isn't always easy. Starting a new business takes time and effort, and the statistics on failure rates suggest the odds are stacked against anyone who tries.

But if you believe in what you are doing—really believe in it—and are willing to work, you can succeed.

Here's some advice: Be fair to your employees at all times, keep learning by reading everything you can get your hands on, and use a lot of common sense.

I strongly believe in the balanced life.

Eat healthy, work hard, have fun.

Loving heart.

Use your thinking rights.

I think Michael McDermott, who wrote an article about Seattle Sutton's Healthy Eating in the magazine "Creative Business," posed the question well.

"We are all hopeful of finding positive answers to the questions: Are there any honest businesses run by honest people? Can one build a successful company on the principles of treating your customers and your employees fairly, and delivering on what you promise?"

McDermott's answer was a resounding "yes." He pointed directly at us.

We agree.

We did it. We are still doing it.

I'm happy when people notice.

Creating a company from scratch—especially one dedicated to helping people—is one of the greatest pleasures of life. I believe it has religious and spiritual relevance, because, after all, we are made in the image of a Divine Creator.

That's why it's important, when bringing an idea into the world, to avoid the error of thinking it belongs exclusively to you. A "creation" has to be raised, and nurtured, like a beloved offspring. Overprotection is a mistake.

Trying to control every aspect of an emerging idea—or child—is not the best creative path, and forces even the most freedom-loving person to rely on "control" techniques which detract from the actual and potential beauty of the unfolding concept.

Actual delegation of authority, on the other hand, is trust in action.

When I started, I had no experience, and no model. Which gave me no preconceptions, and thus the freedom to use my thinking rights.

Other people were drawn to the company, and became part of the creative process. Day by day we made progress.

Being "who we really are" led us to develop a business plan which succeeded in the marketplace, and allowed us to make decisions consistent with what we consider the "right way."

To put it bluntly, the money part of the equation has to work so we can pay our bills and survive. But we handled that in the design, and not being greedy (which means in this context, "not making profit the sole basis of our corporate policy"), we tend to make decisions according to criteria that many companies run by men would most likely not value.

At Seattle Sutton's Healthy Eating, we are nurturers who believe in fair play. Our primary values were established in 1985, and have not changed one iota. "Put the customer first, keep our promises."

I'm proud to say we never deviated from those principles.

My vision hasn't changed since 1985. I have tried to benefit as many people as possible. I believe in this objective so strongly that I even sold the company to accomplish it. That didn't work!

The whole point is to bring healthy eating to as many people as possible. This goal is more important than ever. The current generation does not want to cook, and the next one won't know how.

As a consequence, the Home Meal Replacement (HMR) market has grown rapidly in the last ten years, and is now yielding more than $70 billion annually.

From the day I strolled into Kathy and Dick Naretty's back yard party holding a copy of the Wall Street Journal, I believed in the inevitability of HMR growth.

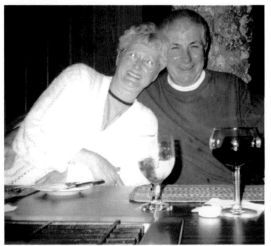

Kathy and Dick Naretty

Anyone who fancies that people will return to their kitchens and cook their own healthy, portion-controlled meals is dreaming. It's not going to happen.

Additionally, aging and overweight baby boomers are searching for healthier choices. Quality—and length—of life are excellent motivators.

Guess what? We believe our company, run by four women, has become the world's leader in healthy eating home meal replacement.

In January of 2002, we moved into a brand-new 25,000 square feet facility that cost the four owners $2.3 million.

It's satisfying to look back at our previous three locations, and see how we have been able to apply knowledge gained from experience to upgrade each facility from its immediate predecessor.

Our new location has a meal-production capacity of approximately 500,000 a week. Since our current high is right at 150,000 per week, we have room to grow, and can use some of our excess capacity to help launch franchises in neighboring states.

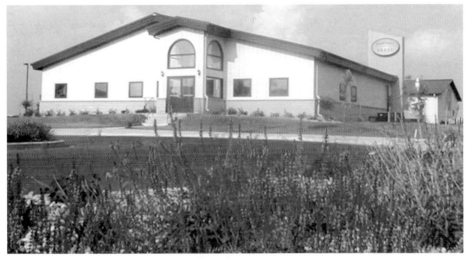

Headquarters

Our new facility—nearly five times as large as our previous—is built on 4.5 acres just north of I-80 in Ottawa, Illinois.

Our old building was only 5,000 square feet, and had little space for parking. Now we have 25,000 square feet and parking for all our employees, and trucks. The design is one large building with about 80% production area (including ample storage), and 20% office space.

It's the first time we've had enough room. Wonder how long that will last?

Kathy Tuntland told the Ottawa Daily Times that we chose to stay in the area because the people "have a good work ethic" and our company is run by "home-town" people.

We own eight huge refrigerator trucks. We started by leasing, and then, as these leases expired, bought new trucks outright. For cash, of course.

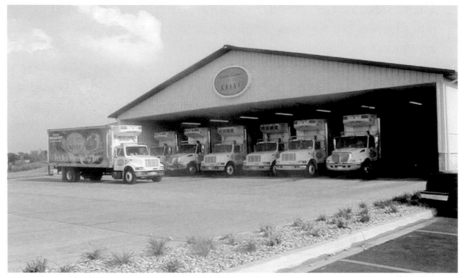
Seattle Sutton's Healthy Eating delivery trucks, circa 2004

Kathy deserves the kudos for our new building. I was never present when she met with the architects and planners.

Kathy asked, "Seattle, don't you even want to look at these plans?"

"Not really."

"But I'm worried. What if I make a mistake?"

"Don't worry Kathy, if needed, we'll move a wall."

When the building was finished, and we had been operating in it for about three weeks, I asked her, "Do we need to move any walls?"

She looked at me kind of surprised, as if reprising our original conversation. Then she answered: "No, we don't!"

So that's the confidence I have in her, though she previously had never designed a building. I knew she would use her thinking rights!

Franchising poses a dilemma for our company. Kathy and I have always agreed we will never jeopardize our company to do nation-wide franchising.

We are working to integrate our business philosophy with an acceptable franchising program. How can we maintain quality? That is absolutely essential. How can we maintain our first-rate employee-management relationship? We have no interest in creating an uncaring monster of a company.

Our employees are happy, our customers are happy, our suppliers are happy, and we owners are happy.

We don't have to worry about pleasing our investors.

We are our investors.

Expansion is a part of our vision, because it meets our goal of bringing healthy eating to more people, but the process has to be well-considered, and carefully managed.

New people are seeking to be involved, and it's important that they earnestly and honestly desire to operate by our principles. If they don't, greed will enter the equation, and that's the wrong way to grow.

We're certainly not interested in "battling" our franchisees over issues like menu choices, or selling a client fewer than 21 meals a week. Yes, we're picky, and not in any hurry.

Which gives us opportunities to carefully assess potential buyers. Kathy and I make it a policy to be open and honest with applicants, and we expect the same from them. That's why we sell our own franchises.

We're looking for good people who keep their promises, and are willing to manage their franchise in a manner consistent with our principles.

Most franchises cover an entire state, but California will end up with three, and Florida and Texas with two each.

Franchisees pay $35,000 plus 5% royalties, and will invest a total of about $1.0 million to build and staff their own kitchen and delivery facilities, and advertise the product.

In some nearby states, as mentioned, we are willing to let the franchisee buy meals made in our Illinois kitchen. For example, we make the meals for our Michigan franchise owner, Wallace Duvall. Our trucks deliver to the southwest corner of his state, where Wallace takes over the transportation and supplies his distributors.

He plans to eventually open his own kitchen in suburban Detroit. Until then we're able to use our kitchen to make it quicker and easier for him to get rolling. That same process might be useful in some other nearby states.

Since the basis of franchising is "selling" the company's name, philosophy, and procedures—and our name has come to denote integrity and excellence—we are exceptionally careful.

We had the luxury of developing the company very slowly, so we were able to avoid debt. Our franchisees are going to have debt, because they are moving faster, racing toward and beyond the break-even point. We need to be sure an applicant can handle the challenge.

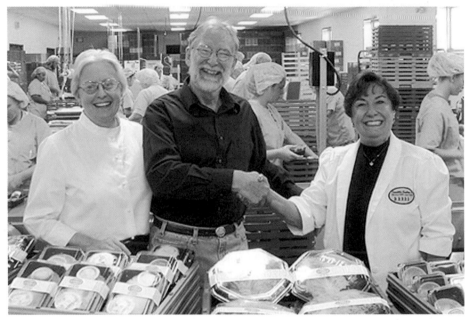

Sarah Burmeister and Chris Gyoury, our Georgia franchisees, visit our headquarters kitchen

One well-known franchising consultant said publicly that our "expansion would be easier if we separated franchisees' marketing and distribution duties from wholesale food preparation." He is of the opinion that we could "significantly improve our ability to sell franchises" by targeting people who run commercial commissaries.

I don't think so.

So far I have rejected franchise opportunities with food industry professionals, perhaps because of my experience with Freshly Yours. And I've turned down venture capitalists who want to invest in a franchise. I simply prefer that investors be involved in daily management.

We receive a large number of franchise inquiries, but if we don't think the people are right, we tend to weed them out very quickly.

Americans now spend about $40 billion a year to lose weight, so entrepreneurs are interested. But we will not affiliate with people whose sole goal is to make money. We want those people who share our dedication to giving our customers results.

Chris Gyoury and Sarah Burmeister decided to purchase and

operate a franchise in Georgia. We have gotten to know Chris and Sarah very well, and are very glad to have them join us.

Here are a few excerpts from a letter they sent to us:

"Please find enclosed the signed Franchise Agreement along with our check for $35,000. There is one comment we would like to make regarding the contract.

"Sarah and I are entering into this agreement guided by our personal assessment of Seattle's exceptional fairness and practicality in developing this line of business. She has gathered around her key personnel in whom we also place our trust.

"In short, our investment is, for all practical purposes, in her, and it is imperative that, should the company change hands and the franchise agreement be assigned in the future, (it) continue as much as humanly possible with the same high standards and conduct that we have come to know.

"Please note we are not asking for any amendments to the contract… and simply want our concerns…to be noted."

Duly, with gratitude and appreciation.

Sometimes I wish the information we give to our franchisees, like recipes, labeling, ingredient acquisition, preparation and packaging techniques, delivery, distribution management, advertising, etc., would have been available to us in the beginning.

Of course, that's not possible. We developed expertise over time, using our thinking rights, and trial, error, and refinement.

We discovered what works okay, what works fine, and what works best. Looking back, it was fun, because all of us were on the same page, and learning together.

By the way, the $35,000 franchise fee includes training we give at our headquarters. We train every key person, including advertising managers, refrigerated truck drivers and loaders, distributor management, grocery purchasing, meal preparation, and packaging personnel.

We teach labeling, and ordering. We—and our franchisees—don't need inventory because we know the meal rotation and can plan ahead. The only thing that changes is the number of orders.

Given our ability to buy in precise and predictable amounts, we are able to avoid waste. Definitely helps keep our costs down.

I know that other companies trying to copy our approach don't accept this philosophy. Maybe that's why some have had to charge their customers three times as much.

By now, you probably realize that I have a distaste for waste, and it's only natural that the business should reflect my thinking.

A franchise owner has to have refrigerated trucks, employees, insurance, a kitchen, restaurant equipment, and more. We estimate the total cost to get ready for meal delivery to be approximately $750,000.

Plus we suggest an initial advertising budget of $250,000. I believe the only way a franchise can fail is if the advertising is insufficient.

So that's why we predict a start-up cost of one million.

Of course, the next challenge is surpassing a break-even point. To do that, food preparation has to be carefully managed, which mostly means developing appropriate staffing levels.

How can a franchisee recover their million dollars?

By working hard.

And by being dedicated and trained to do the "Seattle Sutton" thing the right way.

We sent two supervisors to Minnesota recently, and they came back delighted because that state's franchise owners, Stephanie Keegan, and her husband, Jim, had put a system in place that produced meals that looked—and tasted—exactly like ours.

Stephanie believes that selling Seattle Sutton's is not "like merchandising a pair of jeans that can be pulled off a rack. We are building a brand from the ground up. That is a challenge we anticipated."

It's kind of interesting that our new franchises are having so many potential distributors inquire for territory even before they go into production. In Georgia, for example, a preliminary meeting resulted in 20 very good distributors.

As soon as it became known that we had established a franchise in Michigan, many of our Illinois distributors contacted their friends and relatives. I think virtually every distributor in Michigan so far originated via an Illinois contact.

This speaks well of our distributor manager. She's my daughter, as you may remember.

My mother, at age 91, visited Ottawa at the time of our 2002 annual distributor gathering, and we asked her to speak. Like any daughter, I want to please my mom. So I was very curious what she might say. I asked, but she refused to tell me. I think she enjoyed keeping a secret from me.

My curiosity did not abate. I felt like a young girl on Christmas Eve, wondering about presents that couldn't yet be opened.

Finally the day of the meeting arrived. We moved through the agenda until the time arrived for Mom to take the podium. She surveyed the audience, smiled, and spoke.

"I'm very proud of Seattle and what she has accomplished. The new building is complete and it is beautiful. Thank you all of you for helping her, because without you she would not be here today.

"Seattle has nothing bad to say about anyone. I asked her, 'Where do you find all these good people?' and she answered, 'There are still a lot of good people in the world.' It's unfortunate we usually only hear about the bad ones."

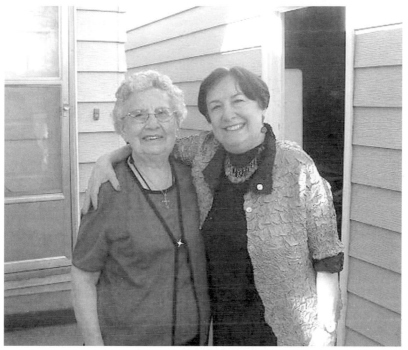

Mother and Daughter

Hurrah for my Mom. I followed her to the podium and told our distributors, "I worried about what she might say because she refused to tell me. On principle."

That generated a round of hearty laughter.

In 2003, I was named a finalist in Ernst & Young's "Entrepreneur of the Year" competition in the category, Illinois Retail and Consumer Products. I didn't win the big prize. But I was pleased that our company's values had earned the respect of the independent judges who selected the finalists.

In the era of World Com, Enron, and many other corrupted bean counter companies, I felt our company had earned some very real respect.

I did receive the statewide Entrepreneurial Success Award, given by the Governor of Illinois, in 2002.   I consider this honor to be an affirmation of the viability of our "small town" approach to business.

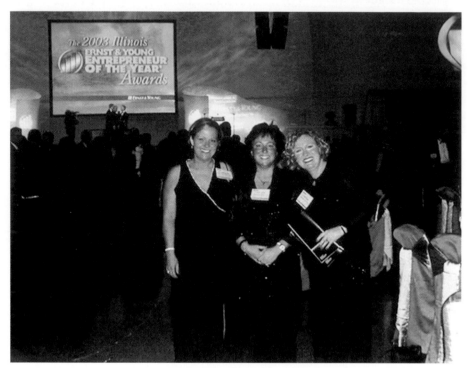

**Sarah, Ruth, and Paula supporting me
at the Ernst & Young dinner**

Chapter Nineteen

We operate Seattle Sutton's Healthy Eating by a philosophy counter to the modern management strategies used by too many companies.

The idea that we should be ruthlessly competitive within our own ranks seems preposterous to me. A player on a basketball team who doesn't cooperate with her or his teammates is called "selfish" and "a cancer."

I also think that anyone who describes "survival of the fittest" as the basic law of commerce hasn't learned very much since leaving the jungle.

Our company is small town, and our business is headquartered in one. As I've mentioned, we started from scratch, and consistently operated by our own values, not the "general modern business" approach.

In the beginning, this added to our degree of difficulty. Who cares? The greater the challenge, the greater the satisfaction.

So what if most businesses attempt to achieve their goals "motivating" employees and managers by competition, punishment, discipline, and fear?

To be clear, let me report that all four owners very much like and admire men. We're all happily married. We're not militant feminists.

Goodness, we're not even non-militant feminists. We're successful people—women—with opinions of our own.

I don't like it when I see a woman trying to be a male. I love guys but don't want to be one. Being female is wonderful.

Women are capable. Women can do! Especially in the entrepreneurial.

We love our husbands, though we often sit back and laugh about the fact we don't believe that they—or maybe any other four men—could have grown our business and made a success like we have.

Men can do some things better than women, but that doesn't include developing businesses like ours.

Why? Here are a few reasons.

First of all, some women work harder than some men. That's a fact. Try raising children if you don't agree.

Also, females, in general, are superior multitaskers. If an emergency arises, and we have to make a quick decision, we can do that while monitoring something else.

Most of us are not afraid—or too proud—to ask for help.

To be more specific, at Seattle Sutton's, we follow a straight and true guideline: find the right solution to a problem, apply it, and don't worry.

That's right. We don't have to build an "it's not my fault" wall to protect us in case of failure.

We make decisions. We don't look back. If it turns out we were right, we're happy; if wrong, we adjust.

Everyone is human. Everyone makes mistakes. We're all pretty forgiving. That comes from the top down.

Ruth, Kathy, Sarah, and I purposely and naturally have built an atmosphere of psychological safety—a comfort zone, if you will, where people know there's not going to be any bickering. And there isn't.

We approach problem solving by "being open." One can't say dismissively about a suggestion or complaint, "Well, this isn't good for us, or the way we do things, and that's it."

Openness unlatches the gate and shows the path. Listening—really hearing—all sides of a problem is the correct route to the right solution.

An environment where everyone feels free to speak honestly and directly is highly desirable.

Don't hide your feelings. Expect the same from others. Think, and say what you think. The problem's solution will present itself.

If we notice a valued employee is in difficulty, we try to help. We don't do this for ulterior, Machiavellian goals—although our company is well served by generating loyalty. We do it because that's what we think is right.

In short, we believe in taking care of each other. Not surprising, because women, as a group, are more nurturing than males. I think men are more interested in the bottom line, and progressing their career.

Of course, this is a generalization, and I have known many supportive males, including my father and husband and sons, and Kathy Tuntland's husband, and Sarah's, and Ruth's, and Paula's, and many, many, many, more.

If they hadn't been there for us, we wouldn't have been able to grow Seattle Sutton's into the success it has become. I guess the truth about gender is undeniable. We need each other.

Success creates many opportunities to teach. I think it's right to step up to the plate as much as possible. Yet I was nervous when an instructor at Lewis College asked me to address his graduate marketing class.

Never having taken a marketing course, I didn't know what to expect. But I have a direct manner, so, putting aside any concern, I strolled to the podium, and started to speak.

I told the students that the ideas I used to start our innovative company didn't come from a marketing manual. They came from within and were an expression of the life I have lived.

How did I learn to manage a business? By being a parent of five children.

Parenting takes work and planning. I had to stay a step ahead, so I learned to anticipate problems, and try to find solutions. This practice paid dividends later.

I gave the grad students an example.

Problem: I wanted to reward and support my most successful distributors, but I didn't want to give them a trip to Las Vegas, or something like that, where they would just spend their money—and be away from their phones. I needed something that would assist them and promote business.

Solution: A plan to honor our best distributors by name, and trumpet their success in our weekly, "News and Clues" letter. And I give them bonus dollars to use for local advertising, which headquarters pays directly to their chosen media company.

Simple and to the point. But as I described it, a light ignited in the students' eyes. I could feel their spirits rousing to life! Someone was encouraging them to use their thinking rights!

Soon the questions were flying. They asked my advice to help them succeed, and (I'm sure by now you're not surprised) I gave it.
- Be honest, patient, and willing to work more than 9 to 5
- Be fair to the people with whom you work.
- Have a positive attitude.
- Pay attention to detail.
- Return telephone calls promptly.
- Listen to other people's viewpoint.
- Avoid arguments and grudges.
- Forgive and forget minor infractions.
- Do as much as you can as far in advance as possible.
- Keep accurate, well-organized notes.
- Delegate as much as practical.

(The secret to delegation is evaluating the skills of the people involved. Can this person handle the job? Grow and continue growing? Be loyal? The thoroughness of an upfront evaluation is essential. Once a delegation is assigned, and is not successful, well, then you have a real problem.)

- Share profit fairly.
- Resist the temptations of greed.
- Pay bills promptly.
- Do better than expected.
- Show respect to all.
- Appreciate your job.

I assured the students that, although the "share profit" approach may result in less money for ownership, it always generates more happiness for all.

Common sense tells us that the greatest asset people have in life is good health. Not a new car or new home. Not a bulging bank account.

Many go through life thinking, "Oh, if I could just buy 'that,' then I would be very happy." Not true. Bought things don't always equate to happiness.

What does? Friendship. A loving relationship. A generous spirit.

Of course I have noticed that it's very difficult to be happy when you don't have enough money to pay the rent or feed the children. A basic level of supply is necessary for peace of mind. There is nothing immoral about earning money.

I believe that most people involved with Seattle Sutton's Healthy Eating develop a sense of "belonging." This identification cannot be faked or purchased.

It is more than good will; it is cooperation and trust, which, as the project progresses, demonstrates the power of unity in motion.

Ownership may say that investing dollars in a company is a risk, and deserves a just reward. Absolutely true!

But it is also a risk to take a mortgage, buy a car, and raise children. To say that venture capital takes the greater gamble is not necessarily true.

Employees, and in our case distributors and franchisees, also have something vital at stake—a life of labor—and should be rewarded by something other than a minimum portion.

Neither labor nor capital should be over or under rewarded. We should help each other live happily. I am serious. This needs to be a priority.

The type and quality of interaction between ownership and employees has a big impact on productivity, self-esteem, and happiness. Life is organized around work. Where we live, our daily routines, our leisure, our schools, our churches, all revolve around our workplace.

Our work environment shapes our sense of the world, and deeply affects our psychological response to the events of our life.

Can a company with 100,000 employees replicate our environment? If not, maybe that company is just too big.

While the unionization process was absolutely necessary because pre-union ownership had a strong tendency to be grossly unfair and abusive, we are now ready to enter another era, for which I believe Seattle Sutton's Healthy Eating can be a model.

Sound idealistic? Yes, it is. But don't tell me it can't be done, because we did it. So can you, dear reader, whether you are an owner or an employee.

Jesus: "Whatever you wish that men would do to you, do so to them; for this is the law and the prophets."

Critics may argue: "Well, that's easy for you to do, because of the way your company is designed."

True. That's the point. We did it on purpose. We organized ourselves in harmony with our best sense of how to succeed, and treat people right.

Did you know that only 13% of Fortune 500 companies have women on their board of directors? Too bad. They need us!

I'd like to reiterate that three of our owners are nurses. That's important. Ruth used to work at Saint Anthony's Hospital Emergency Room in Crown Point, Indiana. Sarah was a pediatric nurse at Silver Cross in Joliet, Illinois. And, of course, I worked in my husband's practice.

(For the record: My other daughter, Paula, is a nurse at Baylor Hospital in Grapevine, Texas. Also, my granddaughter, Erin, begins her nurse's training soon. I hope she plans on being a leader in the "Let's Go Back to Wearing Nurse's Caps and Looking Professional" movement. But who knows? She's been raised to make her own choices.)

I very much enjoy my partnership with Ruth and Sarah. Did you know that neither one has ever complained to me about the other? They work together beautifully. I so admire and appreciate this.

I own stock in many companies, and so do my children, and grandchildren. I understand the value of profit, but I also value happiness. I want both for the members of my family. And yours.

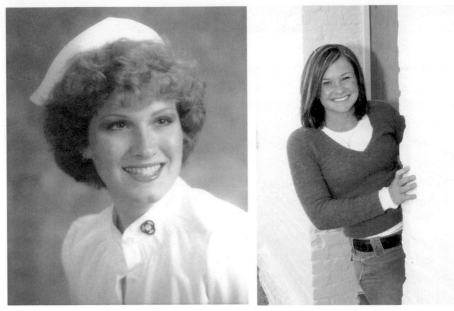

Paula   Erin

Building a business is a struggle, true. Making it consistent with a personal vision requires an even more rigorous and extensive application of willpower.

The process is simplified by the discovery of allies, who show up in unanticipated locations and unexpected ways. It's almost as if a right idea reaches out from our mind to probe the physical universe, seeking friends, allies, answers, and resources.

My original conception—born in 1985—remains a dear and loyal companion. By sticking to my principles, I return its loyalty and guard its borders.

To do so requires perseverance and strength. I give all I have, in my own way, as a natural extension of my true personality.

That is why my business is successful and my life is happy.

I earnestly desire the same for you.

Chapter Twenty

Iwrote this book for you, my dearly beloved grandchildren, so you would have a lasting record of my philosophies on a variety of topics, including healthy eating, parenting, marriage, values, and how to run a business.

I hope you will read it many times, and share it with your children, and theirs. In my imagination, I see you all. This vision makes Kelly and me deeply happy. The idea that a part of us will be present for our future generations pleasures our souls.

One of our church hymns sums up the basic philosophy of Grandpa Kelly and Grandma Seattle: "Love, laugh, and live."

It's true I am old, but I want you to know that I never actually dated Abraham Lincoln. Yet I think I represent the kind of Illinois he helped shape.

We're better educated now than in his time, and our quality of life has improved. If people of good will use their energy wisely, and with compassion, our world will be even better when you are grandparents.

Here's a fundamental truth. Humans can learn. Humans can think. Generation after generation. These are not abstract generalizations, these are your inalienable traits.

Accumulation of knowledge and ability to process information are the chief distinguishing characteristics of our species. I urge you to use your ideas, experiences, and energy to benefit your family as well as yourself, and as many other people as opportunity grants.

I have always been energetic. I like to "do things."

Now that I am older, it is with great satisfaction that I recall a high school science lesson: Energy is never destroyed, it is only changed. I take this to mean my energy will never be destroyed. Nor, thank God, will yours.

How will you use your energy? Those decisions are yours, and no one has the right to take them from you. That's correct.

Nobody can live your life for you. No one else can choose who you will marry, what career you will follow, where you will live, how you will think.

Is anything more precious than these freedoms? I think they are ours because we "are made in the image" of a totally free God.

The best service I can provide my "born free" grandchildren is well-considered counsel. My values and understandings are in part derived from those of my parents and grandparents, and Kelly, and also culled from my long and happy life.

Attitudes and habits pass from generation to generation. If you treat your parents well, and your children see that, chances are they will do the same for you.

Kelly and I take great satisfaction from the respect our children and grandchildren show us, and the respect we have for your parents and each of you. It also makes us very happy that you love to visit us.

By the way, here's a piece of advice that might be useful for you in thirty or forty years. When your grandchildren come to your home, make sure they enjoy their visit. It's important they feel welcome and loved. So if they break a vase, for example, tell them, "I'm so glad because I didn't like it very much."

My dear grandchildren, the ultimate objective—and achievement—is to be happy. Selfishness is not a path to happiness. Love and compassion are the right roads.

All the people I know who are really happy have made a difference in the lives of other people. They have helped the less fortunate, and they have lived courageously, unafraid of distinctive self-expression. As a result, they have brought many excellent ideas into our world.

Don't be overly critical of other people. Your negativity bounces back on you. If I hear someone running down someone else, I think, well, I want to form my own opinion. I don't accept third-person negative judgments.

I think there is good in everyone. If you visited skid row on Madison Avenue in Chicago, and became acquainted with a homeless drunk in the gutter, you could discover many good qualities. It's a matter of perspective.

You can rise every morning and be as miserable and negative as you choose, or you can think positive and be happy, if that's what you prefer.

You have the right and freedom to think negatively, but why not choose a positive attitude? I highly and totally recommend it.

I feel sorry for anyone that feels they gain something by constantly proving that some negativism of theirs is true. Talk about a self-fulfilling prophecy. What a sorry and unhappy state of mind.

When you find problems in your family, your church, your community, your workplace, your country, you should step in and attempt to improve the situation.

Beware the nonchalant person who is always late and missing deadlines. That's not the road to success, even though some people might equate nonchalance with happiness. This is foolish.

I counsel you to be organized and energetic. Make a plan, and fulfill its requirements. Adjust as necessary. Keep moving forward.

When you have a right idea, and are committed to it's successful development, pursue your goal with all your might, and don't worry about the possibility of failure.

Don't be afraid to think for yourself. Don't be afraid of being criticized.

Simply by being willing to try, you have already achieved an important success. If you really believe in something, do it! Remember your grandmother and her late-life business!

Too many people fill their days with worry. If you can't correct or at least address a problem, maybe it's not worth obsessing about.

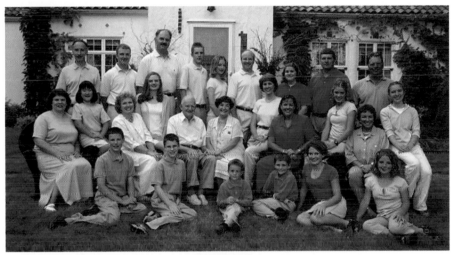

Our family

When Kelly and I first were married, I used to worry about some trivial thing or another, and he told me, "One hundred years from now, who is going to care about that?" He helped me realize that most things aren't worth the wasted energy of worry.

There is a difference between worry and concern. Concern is an attribute of love, but worry is the child of fear. So, to quote Bobby McFerrin, "Don't worry, be happy." Sound advice, my dears.

I greatly value the importance of being able to cooperate in an atmosphere of confidence and trust. Such cooperation is a key element of happiness and success.

I don't fathom why people—and countries—can't get along. Perhaps it's because of a lack of communication. I think the world would be better if we only had one language.

It's easy to study a situation from your own perspective. It's important to study it from the viewpoint of the other fellow. Remember the story of Sarah and her stolen bike.

Religion is another area of unnecessary division. I don't believe any one church is better than any other. So I don't think people of one religion should criticize another.

The reason we have so many churches is because human beings have conceived many different interpretations of a basic truth, and too many times someone insists on codifying an insight into a dogma.

Religions can be very different, and it is the right of all people to worship as they please, but we all have the same God. We all need to be good to one another and lead a right life.

A more significant distinction is between those who believe in God, and those who don't. And even this difference does not suggest the necessity of a lack of cooperation, or a feeling of superiority.

God takes care of all of us, and I just can't imagine a failure to accept one or another belief system as just cause for some sort of ultimate punishment. This seems far more a human concept than a divine one.

Trying to control others—in the family and/or at work and worship—is a serious error. Besides, it can't be accomplished without resorting to techniques that infringe on free choice and fair play—and that's a form of evil.

Allow me, dear grandchildren, to change the subject to one of my favorites. You might think that right now I'm going to write: "Calories in versus calories out." My fondness for this excellent maxim is well-known. And I did write it, so I guess you were right.

But this is what I really intended to say: Keep the body healthy by giving it the right fuel. Never forget this truth—no matter how strong the temptation.

Putting the right portions of the right foods into your mouth is essential for happiness. Eating right helps keep you healthy, and, without good health, how can anyone be happy? How can anyone achieve a goal?

I'm going to share with our readers the contract Kelly and I have with our grandchildren. Here is an excerpt from our most recent Christmas letter to each of you:

"Our gifts to you: You now own 50 shares of Agilent Technologies, Inc. The purchase price was $26.92 per share, so $1,346 was added to your Charles Schwab College Account. Also:

$100 cash. And a video celebrating Seattle Sutton's Healthy Eating to save for your great grandchildren.

"Your gifts to us: You will never smoke because it will ruin your body. You will not drink alcohol until age 21 (and then only in moderation). You will not go steady in high school because you are not yet ready to make a marital choice.

"You will not put rings in your nose, belly buttons, tongues, etc. to embarrass us. You will treat your parents as you will someday expect your children to treat you. You will attempt to do your best in school, including college. You will continue to show respect to others, and your country.

"Managing your money: We expect you to be financially savvy. Never make a charge on a credit card unless you have the money necessary to pay the charged amount "in full" as soon as the bill arrives. If you get into the "minimum payment" trap, you are in a financial self-destruct mode. We ask you to avoid it by not spending money you don't have.

"Live within your means. Don't let anyone encourage you to get into debt. When you get your first job, save some money from every paycheck. In other words, pay yourself first before spending on anything. Small amounts grow to tremendously large sums over time. The sooner you start saving the better!"

Yes, that's our contract. More is expected, so more is given.

Our arrangement is designed to protect you against making bad decisions while you are young. The quality of an entire life is often decided during these formative years. Kelly and I are simply looking at the "big picture" and doing what we can to be helpful guides.

One of the worst dangers you face is negative cynicism. You are not alone. Too many are in peril of losing faith in the power of idealism, which is a vision of something better, and a hope that this improvement can be brought into the material world.

Don't lose your faith, my wonderful grandchildren. A "practical" perspective has to be rooted in the earth, but also requires the boldness of wings.

When you need an antidote to defeat cynicism, I suggest you remember the "village values" so vital to your parents and Kelly and me.

Small town people nurture their neighbors, treat people fairly, and know the difference between right and wrong. It's an excellent way to operate, even if your lifestyle does not give you the opportunity to make a home in a smaller community. Wherever you find your-

self, do your best. As I said to my Mother, good people are every-
where.

My beloved grandchildren, I ask each of you to live a heroic life.
How do I define such a glorious path?

By taking my cue from Joseph Campbell, who wrote:

"The hero is the one who comes to participate in life courageously and decently, in the way of nature, not in the way of personal ran-
cor, disappointment, or revenge."

God bless you one and all.

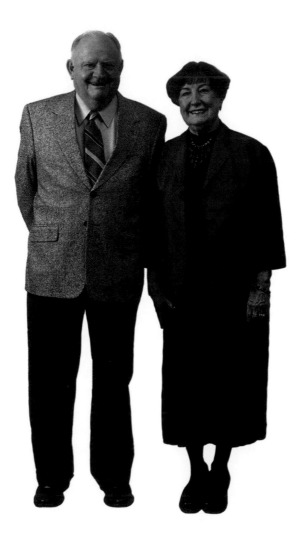

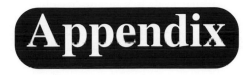

Appendix

Acknowledgements

I would like to acknowledge and thank the many good people who have helped me in my life, my business, and with this book. Of course, the trouble with actually compiling a list is the certainty that imperfect memory will inadvertently omit many who merit my wholehearted gratitude.

So let me begin by saying a general "Thank You" to every single one of my friends, neighbors, and allies. Many of you are mentioned in this book.

But the fact that your name may not be present on these pages does not mean it isn't written in my heart.

I wrote this book to provide a testimonial to individual creative power, and the necessity of loving cooperation. I hope you will benefit from reading the story of my life. I have lived it in as loving a way as possible, and I am always learning.

I believe in free choice, honesty, and fair play. In my life and business, I have been able to meet and work with many who share the same beliefs, and steer by the same stars.

The diet industry is full of hype and outrageous claims, and, while Seattle Sutton's Healthy Eating is a right answer, sometimes it can be difficult to discern a solitary diamond in an acre of zirconium.

Without further ado, in no particular order except for the first twenty-two, I'd like to present my acknowledgements and thanks to:

My parents, my husband, my five children, and fourteen grand-children.

Dear friends: Kathy and Dick Naretty. Harold and Helen Danelson. Robert and Marlene Smith. Floyd and Wanda Kingston. Ted and Jane Myrna. Arlene Campbell. Bud and Elaine Spencer. Helen Allen. Ruth Farrell. Wayne and Sharon Alsvig. Maggie Miller. Kathleen Tuntland.

The people of the First Congregational Church of Marseilles, Illinois. Betty Galloway, our church clerk.

Boyd Palmer, director of Illinois Valley Community College's Small Business Development.

Our distributors. What a great group! So many outstanding people!

My niece Bonnie, and her husband, Everett Wieland. My nephew Wendell Janke and his wife Dixie; and my other nephew, Richard Janke.

David Swartz. Tammy Blacklaw. Dave Ostrowski.

Attorneys: Stuart Hershman, franchising; Ed Sutkowski, corporate; and Mike Reagan, local.

All of Seattle Sutton's Healthy Eating employees. Thanks to our truck drivers, packagers, cooks, bakers, preppers, administrators, and all the rest.

My first employees: Rosemary Martin, Carol Macchietto, Sal Clark, Gale Swartz, Mary O'Dell, Pat Kesler, Janice McDonald, Betty Ball, Ray Page, and Gene Panti, who is still with us.

Dr. Muhammad Khan. Laura Farjood, R.D. Bill Spicer. Neda Kane. Paula Holler. Bob Jones. Vivian Crose.

All the people at Twin Oaks Bank in Marseilles. Scott Caselli of Caselli Insurance. Kevin Nordquist. Liz Cullen. Ewa Olejnik. Ann Greitl.

Kelly's poker buddies, who keep him occupied when I don't have a lot of time to entertain him.

I want to take this opportunity to express my gratitude for the fine education I received at Jamestown College, and to thank the supervisors, directors, and instructors at the College and Hospital for their dedication to our education, and their interest in us as developing individuals. Because of them, I have been immeasurably strengthened throughout my life, and their influence continues to this day, up to and including my writing of this book.

Susie Farrell Reusch transcribed my book dictation. Sue Herrin contributed as proofreader and editor. Patsy Brown helped with the proofreading. Dave Swartz assisted in the management of the production process. Harold Clemens and Erik Connelly of ADventure Advertising & Printing printed the book. Their employees, Jeff Miller and Keith Seroka, assisted with the graphic design. By the way, except for Sue, those mentioned in this paragraph are all local people.

This section is definitely not as much fun to write as I thought it might be. I fear I'm forgetting many people. I could include the whole town of Marseilles! And Ottawa. And Gackle. Plus every employee, distributor, and franchisee.

To everyone who's not listed, please accept my apology, and my gratitude. Thank you for being a part of my life.

I'm glad we share the same time and space.